A Comprehensive Hand Book For Traditional Chinese Medicine Facial Rejuvenation

Ping Zhang, Ph.D., LAc.

A Nefeli™ Corporation Publication

Disclaimer: Information contained in this book is given in good faith and is based on Traditional Chinese Medicine teaching and author's experience. The author and the publisher make this information available for Traditional Chinese Medicine practitioners as a source of information for research and scholarly purposes only. It should not be used to diagnose, treat, cure or attempt to prevent any disease and should by no means be considered a substitute for the advice of a qualified healthcare practitioner, who should always be consulted before beginning taking any herbs/herbal supplements, new diet, exercise or other health program. Any application of the material set forth in this book including internal taking and external application of any herbs/herbal formulas, foods suggestions, acupressure routines as well as Qi Gong exercisers is at the reader's discretion and sole responsibility. The author and publisher cannot be hold responsible for any error or omission. Nor can they be held in any responsible for treatment given on the basis of the information contained in this book.

The author and the publisher expressly disclaim responsibility and liabilities for any adverse effects, injuries or damages arising from the use or application of the information contained in this book

Fourth Printing, December 2008   ISBN: 978-1-5997-5666-0

Nefeli Corp., 319 Port Washington Blvd., Port Washington, NY 11050

Visit our website at www.nefeli.com

Printed in the United States of America

PREFACE

This comprehensive handbook for Traditional Chinese Medicine (TCM) rejuvenation covers the complete guide of acupuncture, Chinese herbal medicine, acupressure, Chinese food therapy, Qi Gong exercises as well as other modalities including Gua Sha, Moxa, and Jade Stick massage techniques for facial rejuvenation concerns such as wrinkles, sagging of the face, facial discoloration and age spots, dark eye circles and eye bags.

The book consists of three parts separated into 29 chapters. Part I covers TCM Comprehensive Facial Rejuvenation Protocols. In Part II, Ping Zhang shares her advanced TCM facial rejuvenation protocols with the readers. Some of these materials have been presented in Ping Zhang's professional TCM Facial Rejuvenation seminars and in the classes she taught for Now York College for Health Professions. In Part III, A step-by-step protocol for TCM facial rejuvenation is introduced for those who are interested in set up a TCM treatment spa in their office.

I hope this handbook will add valuable information to your current TCM facial rejuvenation practice so we can help our patients to have a better life and more rejuvenated face from the inside out.

Ping Zhang, Ph.D., LAc., NH., NCCAOM

Contents

Part III

DIY Herbal Shop: TCM Needleless Facial Rejuvenation

Part I

TCM Comprehensive Facial Rejuvenation Protocols

Section 1
Introduction to TCM Facial Rejuvenation

Chapter 1
History of TCM Facial Rejuvenation

The practice of facial rejuvenation therapies enjoys a long and rich history in Traditional Chinese Medicine (TCM). Beginning in the early Western Zhou period (1121–770 B.C.), Chinese healers developed special modalities to treat a variety of skin conditions. These included dietary adjustments intended to heal both physical and mental ailments as well as to prevent disease and combat aging.

The famous text, *Classic of Mountains and Seas* (*Shan Hai Jing*), authored during the Warring States period (770–221 B.C.), itemized over 150 different herbal therapies of which many dealt with facial rejuvenation. The traditional healing therapies and modalities as well as their philosophical underpinnings were later modified during the Han dynasty (206 B.C.–220 A.D.) in the text, *Yellow Emperor's Inner Classic* (*Huang Di Nei Jing*), the most important text in the canon of Traditional Chinese Medicine.

The earliest book legend for traditional Chinese herbal medicine that included facial rejuvenation was *The Divine Husbandman's Classics of Materia Medica* (*Shen Nong Ben Cao Jing*). This seminal text documented over three hundred different therapeutic herbs. The so-called "Superior Herbs" possessed antiaging and facial rejuvenating properties.

Later texts built upon the foundation of Traditional Chinese Medicine by introducing new concepts and techniques. During the Shui (221–256 A.D.) and Jin (265–420 A.D.) dynasties, texts such as *The Systemized Canon of Acupuncture and Moxibustion* (*Zhen Ju Jia Yi Jing*) (282 A.D.) added acupuncture techniques to the existing modalities of facial rejuvenation. Ge Hong, a great Daoist practitioner of the healing arts, developed over thirty unique formulas including herbal masks designed to treat a variety of aesthetic and rejuvenating issues.

Further refinements occurred during the Tang dynasty (618–907 A.D.), the so-called Renaissance in Chinese history. Sun Si Mao, the most famous of all early Daoist physicians, compiled two great texts, *Thousand Ducat Formulas* (*Qian Jin Yao Fang*) and *Supplement to the Thousand Ducat Formulas* (*Qian Jin Yi Fang*), which contributed greatly to the study and practice of rejuvenating therapies. Building upon the existing foundation, Sun Si Mao developed innovative modalities utilizing herbs, acupuncture, and dietary adjustment to find new ways to promote health, longevity, and beauty.

Acupuncture as a means to facial rejuvenation gained even greater recognition during the Song dynasty (960–1280 A.D.). Texts, including *The Life Promoting and Prevention Classic of Acupuncture and Moxibustion* (*Zhen Ju Zhi Shen Jing*) by Wang Wei Yi, documented the practice of specific points and moxibustion.

The Ming dynasty (1368–1644 A.D.) witnessed further progress in the development of rejuvenating techniques. Li Shi Zhen, among the foremost physicians of his day, authored the classic text *Materia Medica* (*Ben Cao Gang Mu*). Linking chapters to specific facial features, Li Shi Zhen addressed the unique treatment requirements of the eyes, nose, lips, teeth, and hair, as well as the more overriding issues of complexion and wrinkles. The book further links the ameliorative properties of certain herbs to specific health and beauty concerns.

Another great work of the Ming dynasty, Yang Ji Zhou's *Great Compendium of Acupuncture and Moxibustion* (*Zhen Jiu Da Cheng*) had a far-reaching effect on the use of acupuncture in facial rejuvenation. Relying upon the clinical experience of other practitioners as well as his experience, Yang Ji Zhou conceived new modalities utilizing acupuncture and moxabustion.

As noted, the development of facial rejuvenating techniques is a centuries-old process that has drawn upon the cumulative experience and wisdom of the great Daoist practitioners. While acknowledging this valued tradition, today's practitioner must utilize this foundation within the context of the modern world. Changes in lifestyles, social morals, and our natural environment itself require an ever-evolving approach to patient care.

Chapter 2
TCM Facial Rejuvenation Theory

2.1 Zang Fu Theory

Traditional Chinese Medicine (TCM) addresses the same organs as Western medicine, yet organizes them in a different fashion. In doing so, TCM describes their functions with greater complexity and finer detail. For example, although Western science believes the function of the kidneys is to collect and discharge urine, TCM further imbues them with the power of storing essence, thereby housing the ability to govern reproduction. Rather than highly individualized parts of the body, TCM thinks of organs as integrated systems that disperse the qi (energy) they generate via channel flow. In this fashion, seemingly distant organs, such as the liver, can have an important impact on facial beauty.

The Chinese recognize five of the organs, namely the heart, liver, kidneys, spleen, and lungs, as being broadly related because of the type of functions they carry out. They are called the Zang or yin organs, and are considered yin in nature because they retain essence. The remaining organs, the stomach, large intestine, gallbladder, urinary bladder, small intestine, and the San Jiao (or "triple burner"), are called the Fu or yang organs. They do not retain essence, but rather process it. They are related to digestion and perform the function of excreting bodily toxins. The seventh organ, the pericardium, is also thought of as a yang organ. The Zang and Fu organs combine to form the twelve main channels, or meridians, that are based on the organs.

During anti-wrinkle therapy, special focus should be placed on the five Zang organs. Each of the five is paired with a Fu organ in function, creating a yin/yang balance of paramount importance.

For our purpose, we will be addressing the organ systems in a very specific manner. The following review will aid you in understanding how TCM views the functions of the five Zang organs within the scope of facial rejuvenation.

The Heart

According to TCM theory, the heart not only rules the blood and blood vessels, but the spirit as well. Thus, the Chinese call the heart "the king of emotions." Anxiety, stress, anger, and frustration all contribute to the formation and maintenance of wrinkles. To target wrinkles as a major concern, one must target the control of emotions. Therefore, many of the anti-wrinkle treatment protocols will serve to calm the heart.

The Fu organ that is paired with the heart is the small intestine. This organ functions to transform pure food into nutrients and impure food into waste. Thus the heart is indirectly involved in digestion.

Facial Implication: The implication for the face follows that weakened heart function can lead to facial swelling and puffiness. Further impairment of the yin/yang function of the heart and small intestine can lead to heart blood deficiency and the formation of wrinkles. On the other hand, if the heart then is disturbed, sleep will be affected, and restless sleep will cause dark eye circles and puffiness of eyes.

The Lungs

The lung system controls respiration, a qi function. Thus it can be said, according to the *Yellow Emperor's Inner Classic*, "the life energy of the heavens connects to the lungs." By combining the air breathed in with food essence and spreading it to the body as a whole (chest qi), the lung system is able to rule the qi of the entire body. The skin and face come under the dominance of lung qi. To insure the proper functioning of the lungs, many of the herbal formulas and other protocols will necessarily be directed to the lung system.

The organ paired with the lung is the large intestine. Its function is to discharge bodily waste.

Facial Implications: Functional impairment in the lung will lead to undernourishment of the skin. This in turn will lead to dryness, wrinkles, and a withered-looking complexion.

The Liver

The liver system is the key to the anti-wrinkle efforts. It is a blood container and flow regulator. The liver plays a major role in the qi flow of all the other organ systems as well, and as such, the liver is closely linked to all the body's organ systems. A disruption in liver function will therefore disrupt qi and blood flow everywhere, including the face.

The liver's Fu partner is the gallbladder. The gallbladder function relates to the mental state of an individual. When this function is in a state of disharmony, decision-making abilities may be seriously affected.

Facial Implications: The stagnation of liver qi often leads to wrinkles, dark spots, and a dusty complexion.

The Spleen

The spleen is also strongly related to facial beauty. The digestive system pertains to the spleen and stomach and is considered the "postnatal sea of energy." The spleen dominates the function of converting food into qi and blood, making its transformation functions of vital importance for facial beauty and total body health. The face ultimately depends on and responds to what is digested and absorbed in addition to the type and amount of foods ingested.

The paired organ of the spleen is the stomach, an organ that receives and decomposes food.

Facial Implications: When spleen qi is deficient, the skin will be undernourished, resulting in a loss of skin tone, sagging, and looseness. If the spleen's ability to control the transportation of fluids is diminished, the face will tend to look puffy, with the possible appearance of eye bags. Pooling of these unclean fluids may also lead to brownish dark spots on the face.

The Kidneys

The kidney system regulates the fluid balance in the body in many ways. The most familiar being its role in extracting excess fluids from the body. It works with its paired Fu organ, the urinary bladder, to discharge the fluid. TCM also sees the kidneys as the storage center for essence, thereby giving it further involvement with growth and reproduction.

Facial Implications: Deficient kidney yin puts one at a risk for developing dark eye circles and age spots. When kidney yang is low, puffiness around the eyes can occur.

When kidney essence is insufficient, aging is accelerated, affecting skin tautness, which in turn causes wrinkle formation as well as thinning of the hair.

Categories of Risks and Benefits

TCM recognizes a large and variable number of factors can affect the body's functioning, leading to wrinkle formation and other facial beauty problems. One category of these risk factors is environmental conditions called the "six evils." It includes conditions such as wind, cold, summer heat, dampness, dryness, and fire.

The potential damage to facial skin from these conditions is easy to see. It is interesting that TCM sees these same conditions as being both *external* and *internal* factors. For example, when heat is viewed as an internal pathogen, the body is seen as having signs and symptoms associated with the characteristics of heat: swelling, redness, and dryness are related to lack of fluids being burnt off. Chinese herbal therapy and other alternative treatments can deal with such problems.

Another category of health risks is the Seven Emotions. These include anger, joy, worry, pensiveness, sadness, fear, and shock. Again, TCM treatments help control facial beauty problems stemming from emotions by treating imbalances in the organ systems that control them.

2.2 The Five Elements Theory

Other categories of phenomena are involved in the body's functioning. One of the most fundamental categories in TCM is known as the "five elements." The Chinese sages of ancient times were keen observers of natural phenomena, just as natural scientists today. Their observations led them to believe that the physical world was a process of change and that all that exists is the result of transformation based on five basic elements—wood, fire, earth, metal, and water. TCM practitioners saw the same five basic elements in the human body. Moreover, they were able to connect each element to a Zang organ, and then connect that pair to all the factors that determine health or disease—color, taste, emotions, and so on.

When TCM relates the five elements to the human body and it's functioning, it should not be interpreted as saying that the body is made out of earth, fire, metal, etc. TCM deals with properties, using its own metaphors to explain the complex interactions taking place in the body.

By finding relationships between organs and elements, and charting their interaction with other categories of health factors, TCM was able to construct an intricate and useful system for explaining how the body works. This ancient basis for medicine has served well throughout the centuries. The following groupings tell how each element is connected with organ pairs, tastes, colors, emotion, environmental factors and seasons, as well as which sensory organ it correlates to (or "opens to" in TCM parlance).

Wood

Organs: liver and gallbladder

Environmental factor: wind

Direction: east

Season: spring

Rules: tendons and ligaments

Emotion: anger

Color: red, green

Taste: sour

Opens to: the eyes

Fire

Organs: heart and small intestine

Environmental factor: heat

Direction: south

Season: summer

Rules: facial complexion

Emotion: joy

Color: red

Taste: bitter

Opens to: the tongue

Earth

Organs: spleen and stomach

Environmental factor: dampness

Direction: internal, center

Season: late summer

Rules: four limbs and the flesh

Emotion: pensiveness

Color: yellow
Taste: sweet
Opens to: the mouth

Metal

Organs: lung and large intestine
Environmental factor: dryness
Direction: west
Season: autumn
Rules: skin and hair
Emotion: grief, sadness
Color: white
Taste: pungent
Opens to: the mouth

Water

Organs: kidney and urinary bladder
Environmental factor: cold
Direction: north
Season: winter
Rules: bones, marrow, and brain
Emotion: fear
Color: black
Taste: salty
Opens to: the ears

From these associations, TCM has been able to identify and confirm treatments for certain conditions over the centuries. For example, if a patient tends to worry a great deal, has a puffy face with a yellow complexion accompanied by eye bags, five elements theory would view that a disharmonious earth element is the cause of the problem. In this element, the presence of dampness may be blocking nutrient and qi flow. Correct acupuncture treatments and proper herbal and food recommendations must take these factors into consideration.

According to the five elements system, five directions correspondent to five seasonal changes:

- In springtime, direction is east. Because there is more wind in the east, liver wind conditions tend to happen during this season, manifesting as Bell's palsy, drooping of upper eyelid, and muscle spasm around the eyelid.

- In summertime, direction is south and is always accompanied by more heat. Conditions such as heart heat manifests as red face and eyes, with sores appearing in the mouth. In the long summer, overwhelming dampness tends to injure the spleen's normal function, leading to skin conditions such as damp-type acne, eczema, and other related damp heat conditions.

- In autumn, dryness in the west tends to injure the lungs. This manifests as skin rashes, acne, dry skin, and wrinkles.

- In wintertime, exposure to wind cold from the north can cause rough and dry skin conditions.

2.3 Qi, Blood, and Body Fluid Vs. Facial Rejuvenation

Qi, blood, and body fluids are the basic materials that form the human body. These basic materials are transformed into body essence through the internal organ system and then distributed into our skin, flesh, and joints through the channel system. Therefore, qi, blood, and body fluids are closely related to the skin, beauty, shape of the face, hair, and general state of being.

Qi Versus Facial Rejuvenation

Only when there is an abundance of and normal functioning of qi, (the life force of our body) can the body maintain a normal physiology. A healthy qi guarantees a radiant face and a healthy body.

A deficiency in qi contributes to a withered-looking complexion and a low spirit. Stagnant qi blocks the normal flow of the blood, manifesting in dark spots and discolorations in the face. Stagnant qi can further cause fluid and dampness retention in the body, which in turn, can cause puffiness of the eyes and face, and unwanted dark-brown pigmentations. If yang qi is deficient, the body will not be able to warm up, producing a pale-colored face.

Lastly, if defensive qi is lacking, the hair and body will lose nourishment, and the skin will appear dry and cracked.

Blood Versus Facial Rejuvenation

Blood has a close relationship with the complexion of the face. Blood moves through the Zang Fu organ and channel system, nourishing and rejuvenating the body as it flows. When the blood is abundant and flows freely, the spirit will be calm, and the complexion will be supple and radiant. If blood is deficient, it will fail to nourish the spirit, skin, hair, and fingernails, and the complexion will suffer as well. Too much heat inside blood will cause the spirit to be agitated and an abnormal redness in the face. Stagnant blood will promote red spots and facial discolorations.

Body Fluids Versus Facial Rejuvenation

Body fluids, in the same manner as blood, nourishes the entire body, including the skin. Abundant body fluids can promote a healthy skin from dryness. A deficiency in body fluids leaves the skin and eyes dry. This dryness makes the face vulnerable to wrinkles. If body fluids are stagnant, it will affect the entire body system including constipation. Water retention in the body can directly affect the appearance of one's face.

Section 2
Acupuncture for Facial Rejuvenation

Chapter 3
Introduction to Acupuncture Facial Rejuvenation

Acupuncture treatment for Facial Rejuvenation can be traced back as far as 2,000 years ago, when it was documented in the *Yellow Emperor's Inner Classic*. It stated in this bible of TCM that there are 12 major channels and 365 luo channels. All the qi and blood from these channels converge at the neck and then continue up to the head and face. Here they penetrate the orifices. For example, the essence and yang qi from these channels penetrates the eyes, enabling them to see, while alternative qi penetrates the ears, enabling them to hear.

The *Yellow Emperor's Inner Classic* also discusses the combined application of acupuncture, herbs, and food for a rejuvenated life, hence a more vibrant face and body. Many of the acupuncture points mentioned in this book serve to regulate the internal system and benefit facial complexion. As it stated in *The Miraculous Pivot* (*Ling Shu*), the 12 channels are the place from where disease arises and from where disease is healed. This ancient medical text clearly states the significance that the channel system has in life.

Acupuncture treatment for the face and body is based on the theory of the channel system. The entire internal organ system is interconnected with the superficial body system, forming a type of network that runs our bodies. Needling a certain channel system can activate the energy flow in that channel system and thus promote blood flow in the entire system of the body.

According to TCM theory, as previously stated, the entire channel organ systems converge in the face, the most yang place in the body. Proper functioning of the body channel system directly affects facial beauty and the aging process. When the internal system is vibrant with abundant qi and blood, the essence becomes sufficient to be distributed anywhere in the body. This belief is the core supporting acupuncture facial rejuvenation. People may not be convinced that the fountain of youth is from the inside out, but imagine if the internal system is aged. A face-lift can make the face look ten years younger, yet without a healthy glow it cannot be considered young and beautiful. It will lack the vitality that can only be obtained from inside out. The book of *Plain Questions* (*Su Wen*) states, "only the upright qi (zhen qi) exists and is strong; then evil disease cannot come in."

Acupuncture facial rejuvenation that is based on the channel system specifically performs the following functions:

1. Promotes free flow of qi and blood and opens the channel system

A good acupuncture technique can efficiently regulate and promote the movement of qi (zang qi), and blood throughout the channels. As *The Miraculous Pivot* (*Ling Shu*) teaches us, "Only when the stagnation is cleared away, can the channels be vented and Yin and Yang be harmonized."

2. Regulates yin and yang

This concept is very important for facial rejuvenation. Facial beauty and rejuvenation depends on a balanced internal body condition. Only in a yin and yang balanced state can the spirit be nourished, allowing for excess nourishment to rise to the head area and nourish the face. If the yin and yang state of the overall body is imbalanced, there is no harmony with which to work, leaving the face vulnerable to a host of conditions.

3. Regulates excess and deficiency

Another function of acupuncture is to regulate excess and deficiency. This is of paramount importance when it comes to facial rejuvenation. When the internal system is at dis-ease, the whole body will show a biased condition to this fact, and it will reflect poorly in the face. For example, if the spleen is deficient with damp accumulation, the face will prove to be puffy with the appearance of eye bags.

When the yang is exuberant, especially in younger people, acne conditions will be prevalent. With correct acupuncture treatment, these unbalanced conditions can be adjusted depending on the type of needle techniques used and point prescriptions chosen.

Chapter 4
Special Channels and Points for Facial Rejuvenation: Functions and Indications

4.1 REN Channel

As the body's "conceptual channel," the REN channel collects the body's yin energy, regulates all the yin channels of the body. It treats problems in the abdomen, chest, neck, head, and face, as well as corresponding internal organ diseases. Many points from the REN channel can be used for the treatment of anti-aging, weight management, and breast enlargement.

The following points are commonly used for facial and body rejuvenation concerns:

- REN6 – swelling of the face, aging, hair loss, withered complexion
- REN4 – weak constitution, aging, lusterless complexion, chronic disease

- REN12 – weak digestion and dampness in middle jiao with yellow and withered complexion as well as dark spots and puffiness of the eyes and face
- REN24 – swelling of the face, wrinkles around the lips

4.2 DU Channel

As the body's "governing channel," the DU channel collects the body's yang energy and regulates all the yang channels of the body. Many of the points from the DU channel treat mental disorders; heat disease; back, neck, and head problems; as well as corresponding internal organ diseases. Therefore, they also treat facial conditions that are caused by organ malfunctions.

The following points are commonly used for facial and body rejuvenation concerns:

- DU10 – releases wind and heat in the skin layers
- DU14 – clears heat, resolves dark spots
- DU4 – promotes lustrous skin, reduces facial swelling

4.3 Large Intestine Channel

The hand yang ming channel (LI) is full of qi and blood. It also rules body fluids. It performs the function of expelling toxins from the body, which is directly related to the healthy condition of skin. This channel also curves around the facial area. Many points from the large intestine channel treat conditions of the head, face, skin, as well as warm febrile disease and weight loss. It plays a very important role for acupuncture face rejuvenation.

The following points are commonly used for facial and body rejuvenation concerns:

- LI4 – facial wrinkles, facial discolorations, sagging eyes, spasm of facial muscles
- LI9, LI10 – promote qi and blood flow to the facial area; clears toxic heat from the skin
- LI11 – facial discolorations and dark spots; red and swollen eyes

4.4 Stomach Channel

The foot yang ming (ST) channel is full of qi and blood. This is the most important channel in the body for acupuncture facial rejuvenation. It strongly promotes skin healing of the face. It has most local points distributed on the face. It treats digestive conditions; face, head, neck, nose and mouth problems; weight problems; and facial-beauty-related concerns. Points from this channel treat dull complexion, facial discolorations and age spots, wrinkles, sagging of the face, sensitive skin, eye bags, and puffiness.

The following points are commonly used for facial and body rejuvenation concerns:

- ST1 – wrinkles around the eyes, eye bags, dark under-eye circles

- ST2 – wrinkles around the eyes, eye bags, dark under-eye circles
- ST3 – wrinkles around the eyes, eye bags, dark under-eye circles, facial sagging, dull complexion, dark spots, facial discoloration
- ST6 – sagging of chin and neck
- ST7 – sagging of chin and neck, age spots
- ST8 – forehead wrinkles, drooping upper eyelid
- ST36 – dull complexion, sagging face, wrinkles due to qi deficiency, eye bags

4.5 Spleen Channel

The spleen channel (SP), paired with the stomach channel, is the base for postnatal energy. Seated in the body's center, its functions of transportation and transformation are crucial for healthy and beautiful skin. It transforms dampness; firms and lifts skin and muscles; improves dull complexion and rough skin; promotes healthy skin tone; and regulates weight problems.

The following points are commonly used for facial and body rejuvenation concerns:

- SP6 – dark and/or age spots, facial discoloration, dark under-eye circles
- SP9 – puffiness of eyes, eye bags, swelling of face, overweight due to dampness accumulation
- SP10 – dark and/or age spots, facial discoloration, dark under-eye circles

4.6 Urinary Bladder Channel

Paired with kidney channel, the urinary bladder channel (UB) performs the function of water excretion. As the longest channel in the body, it passes the face, head, and back all the way to the lower extremities. It corresponds to five Zang organs and six Fu organs, regulates the internal organs system, calms the spirit, and anchors shen, activates local qi and flow in facial area. Many of the corresponding back shu points treat facial rejuvenation concerns that are related to the imbalance of internal organ functions. They regulate the endocrine system, promote weight loss, improve complexion, and clear sensitive conditions.

The following points are commonly used for facial and body rejuvenation concerns:

- UB2 – wrinkles, puffy eyes
- UB12 – sensitive skin
- UB13 – dry and sensitive skin
- UB15 – nourish shen, beautify face
- UB17 – sensitive skin, wrinkles caused by dry skin, dark spots
- UB18 – dry/oily skin, dark spots
- UB20 – dry skin, withered complexion, puffy and sagging eyes and face, early aging
- UB21 – loose facial muscles and sagging
- UB22 – puffy face, sensitive skin

- UB23 – dry skin, wrinkled skin, age spots, dark under eye circles, early aging
- UB43 – withered complexion, sagging face
- UB60 – dark spots

4.7 Kidney Channel

The kidney channel (KI) rules the reproductive system, growth and aging, regulates water metabolism, and water distribution, and governs bones and marrow. Many points in the kidney channel treat dark and/or age spots, facial discolorations, dark eye circles, and wrinkles due to aging.

The following points are commonly used for facial and body rejuvenation concerns:
- KI1 – facial swelling
- KI3 – dry skin, dark and/or age spots, withered complexion

4.8 Liver Channel

The liver channel (LIV) opens to the eyes, rules the blood. Many points in this channel are used to sooth liver qi stagnation, therefore, they treat facial discoloration, dark spots, dry skin, and lusterless complexion.

The following points are commonly used for facial and body rejuvenation concerns:
- LIV2 – lusterless complexion, dark spots
- LIV3 – wrinkles, dark spots

4.9 Gallbladder Channel

The gallbladder channel (GB) regulates the liver and gallbladder, and promotes movement of qi and blood in the facial area. Many points from this channel treat facial beauty concerns locally.

The following points are commonly used for facial and body rejuvenation concerns:

- GB1 – wrinkles around eyes (crow's feet)
- GB14 – sagging eyelid, wrinkled forehead
- GB20 – dry and sensitive skin
- GB31 – sensitive skin
- GB44 – facial sagging

Chapter 5
Special Auricular Points for Facial Rejuvenation

Auricular acupuncture refers to the use of acupuncture needles or other modalities to stimulate certain parts of the ear for the prevention and treatment of disease. Ear acupuncture has had a long history in TCM. Ear acupuncture treatment for a variety of diseases has been documented in the *Yellow Emperor's Inner Classic* during the Han dynasty and in *Thousand Ducat Formulas* by Sun Si Mao during the Tang dynasty.

Many ancient Chinese medicine texts documented the ear to be closely related to the internal organ system via the channel system. Ear points are not only used to treat diseases of the body with respect to the corresponding organ points, but can also be used as a diagnostic tool for body conditions.

Ear acupuncture for facial conditions follows the same philosophy as regular ear treatment. Because there are corresponding points in the ear that relate to certain organ systems, many of which affect the facial area, stimulating these ear points can produce amazing results for facial rejuvenation.

The following ear points are commonly used for facial rejuvenation:

- **Shen Men** – calms the spirit; clears heat; drains fire; used for dark eye circles due to insomnia, lusterless complexion due to emotional stress, itching skin
- **Endocrine** – regulates liver qi; vents the channel and promotes blood flow; expels wind; strengthens lower jiao; used for dark/age spots, facial discolorations, menopausal conditions
- **Face** – vents the channels and promotes qi flow; used for discoloration, dark/age spots, wrinkles, sagging face, and acne
- **Pi Zi Xia** (same point as brain cortex) – regulates the brain cortex; calms the spirit; increases anti-inflammatory effect; reduces swelling; used for discoloration, inflammation, wrinkles.
- **LU** – clears heat; nourishes lung yin; used for itching and wrinkles due to dryness, withered complexion, dark spots, discoloration
- **HT** – calms the spirit; regulates ying blood; used for withered and/or pale complexion, dark eye circles, wrinkles
- **LIV** – soothes the liver; benefits lung qi and gallbladder; promotes blood flow; harmonizes ying blood; brightens the eyes; used for facial rejuvenation of dark/age spots, discolorations, wrinkles, itching, dark eye circles, eye bags due to liver qi stagnation

- **KI** – tonifies kidney essence; strengthens tendons and bones; brightens eyes; aids hearing; used for wrinkles, dark/age spots, sagging face, dark eye circles, eye bags due to kidney yang deficiency
- **SP** – tonifies spleen qi; nourishes skin; generates ying blood; treats dampness; transports nutrients; used for swelling and puffiness, eye bags, sagging, dark spots and discolorations, dark eye circles due to phlegm
- **LI** – clears lower burner; benefits lung qi; used for acne, dark spots
- **SP on the back of the ear** – harmonizes SP and ST; nourishes skin; used for sagging, puffiness of eyes or face
- **LU on the back of ear** – tonifies lung; clears heat; benefits skin and hair; used for dry, withered skin, wrinkles, and acne
- **LIV on the back of the ear** – soothes liver and stomach; promotes blood flow; used for, discolorations, dark/age spots, wrinkles, dark eye circles
- **KI on the back of the ear** – nourishes kidney essence; strengthens bones and marrow; sharpens hearing; used for discolorations, dark/age spots, wrinkles, dark eye circles
- **HT on the back of the ear** – calms the spirit; strengthens heart heat; benefits facial complexion; used for wrinkles, pale complexion

Note: For regular ear points, two or three points can be used in accordance with the patient's condition. It is very helpful to include one of the following points in each treatment: Shen Men, endocrine, Pi Zi Xia.

For focused treatment, choose the corresponding back point of the ear together with the front point. For example, for sagging and puffiness of face, spleen points in the front and back of the ear can be used together for greater effectiveness.

Ear seeds (use the herb Wang Bu Liu Xiang) can also be used as in regular ear seeds protocols. Make sure to have good hygiene to avoid ear irritation.

Section 3

Traditional Chinese Herbal Medicine for Facial Rejuvenation

Chapter 6
Introduction to Traditional Chinese Herbal Medicine For Facial Rejuvenation

Herbal treatment is at the core of Traditional Chinese Medicine. It accounts for more than 75 percent of TCM practice, and is always a major emphasis in any TCM facial beauty program. Chinese herbs are a rich and potent source of healing energy, and their use has been perfected and refined over the last 3,000 years.

In China, herbs are considered gifts of nature. They are used not to "fight" a disease directly, but to enhance the body's natural healing. They balance and regulate internal functions. By doing so, they eliminate the conditions that lead to complexion problems, wrinkles, and eye puffiness.

Herbs are widely used in TCM as topical treatments. They can be applied as masks, washes, and creams. They work directly on the face to restore glow and smoothness.

Unlike Western herbology, where the very word *herb* refers to plants, Chinese herbs also include minerals and even animal parts. The instructions given for choosing and taking herbs will be simple and easy to follow. But be aware that the science behind the functioning of these herbs is complex and sophisticated. Many factors determine an herb's actions. Centuries of observation and fine-tuning are behind the herb choices that are used for facial beauty program.

According to TCM theory, most herbs don't "fight" wrinkles per se. They help the body's self-healing to correct the conditions that caused the wrinkles in the first place. That's much more effective then just attacking a symptom.

How Chinese Herbs Work

Chinese herbs don't work like Western pharmaceuticals. Though the "active" ingredients in an herb can and have been isolated, an herb's effectiveness is not based solely on its ingredients. All the properties of an herb work together in ways that Western science usually cannot explain.

True, many Chinese herbs contain amino acids, proteins, vitamins, antioxidants, and phytochemicals (plant-based nutrients) that Western medicine recognizes as helpful for the skin. There is certainly overlap between East and West. But this doesn't mean that these known factors are the only reasons herbs containing them help the skin. It also doesn't mean that herbs not containing such known factors can't beautify skin. They most demonstrably do.

In short, TCM doesn't analyze herbs by their chemical ingredients. It categorizes herbs by their properties and observed effects. That includes everything from taste and temperature to the organ channel that it affects or enters.

Here are some of the major ways of looking at Chinese herbs:

Herbs by Levels

The oldest Chinese medical literature divides herbals into three levels: superior, middle and inferior.

- Inferior level herbs are used on individuals with special ailments. They can only be taken safely in small doses. They are often quite toxic.
- Middle level herbs are nourishing and are used for short periods, only and in small doses. They are sometimes toxic, and often used in formulas with other herbs that offset their toxicity.
- Superior level herbs are not toxic and are used for long periods of time to treat many different conditions. They are associated with longevity and rejuvenation and are best for general balancing.

Most of the herbs recommended in this book are superior herbs. And the few that aren't superior are not toxic. They are put in the middle level for other reasons.

Herbs by Taste

TCM practitioners have known for a long time that the taste of an herb tells a lot about the kind of action it will have inside the body. There are seven categories of taste:

- **Sweet:** Herbals with a sweet taste nourish the body and skin, and therefore help rectify a number of deficiency conditions that cause dry or wrinkled skin.
- **Pungent:** Pungent-tasting herbs help energy and blood circulation, clearing up qi or phlegm blockage that causes skin rashes and dark spots.
- **Bitter:** Bitter-tasting herbs clear heat and toxins from the body and skin. They are mostly used for skin rashes and acne.
- **Sour and astringent:** Both these tastes are indicative of the herb's function of stopping fluid leakage in the body. They can help stop excessive secretion of sweat and oil in the skin.
- **Bland:** Herbs with a bland taste tend to help the body leach out excessive dampness and water retention. Combined with other herbs, they are helpful in clearing away puffiness and eye bags.
- **Salty:** Salty-tasting herbs can dissolve nodules and calm the spirit. They are often used in herbal formulas for acne conditions.

Herbs by Channel

Herbs usually benefit one or more specific organ systems by "entering" those organs' channels. For skin rejuvenation, five of those channels are most important.

- **Kidney channel:** Herbs entering the kidney channel generally nourish body essence. (Remember that the kidneys are the storage bins for body essence). They can be found in herbal formulas for nourishing the skin. Many of the herbs recommended for wrinkles and age spots work through the kidney channel.
- **Liver channel:** Herbs that enter the liver channel nourish blood and soothe emotions. They are commonly used for facial discoloration and weakened vision.
- **Stomach and spleen channels:** Herbs entering either or both of these paired channels tonify qi (energy) and help the body transform dampness. If the digestive system is weak, qi will be deficient and dampness obstruction often accompanies it. These herbs have important functions for skin rejuvenation. Spleen and stomach herbs are especially effective for aging skin with wrinkles, facial sagging and eye puffiness, including eye bags.
- **Large intestine channel:** Herbs that enter the large intestine channel are usually used to treat skin conditions like acne and eczema.

Herbs by Function

Chinese herbs are also categorized by what they actually do inside the body. There are many categories of herb function. Here are the ones that are most important for herbal beauty treatments:

- **Herbs that release the exterior:** They are usually pungent tasting and enter the lung channel. Many induce sweating, a good example of "releasing the exterior." Many herbs in this category are used for treating facial discoloration, skin rashes and acne, especially if external wind is a factor in the condition.
- **Herbs that clear away heat:** By eliminating excess internal heat, these herbs clean the blood and detoxify the body. Many of them are bitter and cold in nature and enter the stomach, liver or lung channel. They may have anti-bacterial and anti-inflammatory properties and help the body fight infection. For facial beauty, they are used for acne, skin rashes, dark facial spots and redness of the skin.
- **Herbs that drain downward:** These herbs are used to promote bowel movements in conditions of constipation brought on by heat stagnation, food stagnation, or low energy. Most of them enter the large intestine channel. They are often bitter and cold in nature. Caution is needed with herbs in this category because some are very harsh and can weaken the body. Others, though, are safe and are used for heat-induced skin conditions such as acne.

- **Aromatic herbs that expel dampness:** Warm and aromatic herbs that enter the stomach and spleen channel revive spleen function. Their action can penetrate skin and muscle layers, so they are often used externally as herbal creams. Internally they address any skin conditions coming from weak digestion including facial sagging, and puffy eyes.
- **Herbs that tonify the body:** Herbal tonics replenish essence, help to support the healthy body's immune system, increase energy and regulate internal body balance. Their toning (replenishing) action also helps the body's qi, blood, yin and yang. Most tonifying herbs enter the lung, liver or kidney channels. They tend to be sweet in nature. They are excellent herbs for facial beauty and rejuvenation, and they are used for dull complexions, wrinkles, facial sagging, eye bags and dark circles.
- **Herbs that regulate qi:** Harmonizing qi movement is of tremendous benefit in treating dark spots, facial discoloration, dark eye circles, and eye bags. Most of the herbs that treat qi stagnation are warm and dry in nature and enter the lung, liver, spleen, or stomach channel.
- **Herbs that warm the interior:** By nature, these herbs are warm and pungent and enter the spleen or kidney channels. They are used to treat sagging skin and drooping eyelids due to yang deficiency with internal cold. Some can also be used externally to brighten dull complexions.

- **Herbs that invigorate the blood:** These mostly enter the liver and heart channels and vary widely in taste and temperature. They work to promote blood flow and opening channel systems to move qi. As herbal beauty treatments, they're used for treating skin discoloration and roughness, wrinkles, and dark eye circles. No herb in this category should be taken by anybody on blood thinners.
- **Herbs that calm the spirit:** They enter the liver and heart channels, often anchoring the spirit by nourishing heart blood. In TCM theory, the heart is the house of the spirit, and the liver the house of the soul. Some herbs in this category are actually minerals. Calming the mind and spirit, as mentioned, is extremely beneficial for skin beauty.

Herbal Regimen for Internal and External Application

When suggest the patient start with any single herb, he/she can take it daily from 10 days to two weeks. Then rest for several days and repeat the 10–14 day regimen. Keep that on-again, off-again regimen going for a month or two, and then decide if they want to stay with that herb.

Herbal/food masks and washes follow this regimen: use the mask or wash once a day or once every 2 days for one week, then see how the patient feel. If the patient need to start again, they can rest for several days and restart the regimen on and off for one week to 10 days.

An Important Caution Before Taking Herbal Supplements

The herbs recommend to the patients should be safe in normal circumstances for healthy body conditions, but make sure request the patient's medical conditions and medication they are currently taking before suggesting any herb/herbs/herbal formulas. If a patient has any existing medical conditions, or is pregnant, or nursing, or taking any medications you must consult patient medical practitioner before using any herb/herbs/herbal formulas. This is especially important to prevent any herbal/drug reactions. For example, herbs that move the blood can be a problem if the patient is on blood-thinning medication.

As will repeat later in this book, if your patient feels any discomfort or if any allergic reaction occurs after he/she taking any herb, herbs or herbal formula, stop immediately and recommend the patient consult with their doctor(s).

Also, make sure you use only pure, high-quality herbs for your patients that meet or surpass FDA safety requirements.

Caution for Using Herbs or Food for External Skin Care

Sometimes the body can easily get an allergic reaction to something applied externally for skin care. Because of that possibility, please test any herbal or food used externally, including washes and masks, by first applying it to a small area on the patient's inner wrist or the inner part of the upper arm. Leave it on for 24 hours. If any allergic reaction results (such as a rash, redness, swelling, or itching), do not use that herb or food or formula. If there is no reaction, feel free to use it.

Chapter 7
Individual Herbals for Facial Rejuvenation

The following herbs perform many functions. For the purpose of this book, only those functions related to TCM facial rejuvenation are listed, along with specific indications.

7.1   **Fang Feng** (*Radix Ledebouriellae Divaricatae*)
- Clears wind
- Reduces age spots
- Diminishes discoloration
- Diminishes scars, stretch marks (after birth)

7.2   **Bai Zhi** (*Radix Angelicae Dahuricae*)
- Clears sinuses
- Clears wind
- Regenerates flesh
- Lightens discoloration
- Removes toxic smell from body

7.3   **Bai Fu Zi** (*Rhizoma Typhonii Gigantei*)
- Clears internal wind and phlegm
- Guides Qi and blood to the face

7.4   Ye Ju Hua (*Flos Chrysanthemum Indici*)
- Penetrates deep into the skin cells
- Reduces age spots

7.5   Jin Yin Hua (*Flos Lonicerae Japonicae*)
- Clears heat, detoxifies the skin
- Works well with Ye Ju Hua

7.6   Bai Ji Li (*Fructus Tribuli Terrestris*)
- Stops itching
- Soothes skin rash and calms sensitive skin
- Clears rashes from the face

7.7   Dong Gua Zi (*Semen Benincasae Hispidae*)
- Reduces facial swellings
- Brightens the face; helps eliminate dark/aging spots
- Tonifies spleen and clears dampness

7.8   Yi Yi Ren (*Semen Coicis Lachryma-jobi*)
- Clears toxins from the skin
- Makes skin feel silky

7.9   Gan Cao (*Radix Glycyrrhizae Uralensis*)
- Travels through all channels
- Detoxifies the skin, brightens the face

Caution: Gan Cao can increase blood pressure. Patients with high blood pressure need to exercise caution.

7.10   Xiang Fu Zi (*Rhizoma Cyperi Rotundi*)
- Soothes and promotes smooth flow of liver Qi, works as "hormone" regulator
- Protects the skin from UV exposure

- Helps relieve dry skin and wrinkle conditions

7.11   Ginseng (*Radix Ginseng*)
- Helps skin fight the aging process
- Helps prevent wrinkle formation
- Strongly lifts yuan qi, helps lifting sagging of the face
- Beautifies skin and face

Caution: Ginseng may raise blood pressure. Patients with high blood pressure need to exercise caution, especially Korean ginseng and red ginseng.

7.12   Huang Qi (*Radix Astragali Membranacei*)
- Strengthens skin surface, helps prevent wrinkle formation
- Lifts up sinking qi, expels dampness. It helps improve the condition of sagging of the face, eye bags, and facial puffiness.

7.13   Ce Bai Ye (*Cacumen Biotae Orientalis*)
- Promotes hair growth
- Used for alopecia areata
- Clears acne and oily skin
- Cools the blood

The following herbs are considered by TCM to have blood-moving, antioxidant, and anti-aging properties.

7.14   Dan Shen (*Radix Salviae Miltiorrhizae*)
- Has antioxidant effect
- Helps promote qi and blood flow to the face
- Liver Qi stagnation

7.15 **Dang Gui** (*Radix Angelicae Sinensis*)
- Has antiaging property
- Nourishes dry skin
- Promotes blood flow to the facial area

7.16 **Hong Hua** (*Flos Carthami Tinctorii*)
- Promotes blood flow
- Works for dark/age spot
- Nourishes dry skin

7.17 **Tao Ren** (*Semen Persicae*)
- Helps fight wrinkles
- Nourishes dry skin

Caution: These blood-moving herbs should not be given to patients if they are on blood thinner medications.

Chapter 8
Traditional Herbal Formulas for Facial Rejuvenation

There are many Chinese herbal formulas with anti-aging properties that rejuvenate the body and face by addressing the underlining causes. They are documented in many ancient and modern TCM texts. Below are some of these beauty formulas. Many may be unfamiliar to you.

Ming Dynasty Emperor's Secret
Source: *Ming Dynasty Kingdom Secret Formula*

During the Ming dynasty (1368–1644), the emperor told a team of the best healers in the kingdom to come up with a formula that would rejuvenate his face and prolong his life. After much hard work, they created a formula that pleased the emperor. It consisted of the following herbs, most of which you will recognize from the previous chapter:

- Xian Shen Di Huang (*Radix Rehmanniae Glutinosae*) (fresh rehmannia juice) 10 portions
- Korean ginseng 1 portion
- Gou Qi Zi (*Fructus Lycii*) 1/2 portion
- Tian Men Dong (*Tuber Asparagi Cochinchinensis*) 1/2 portion

- Mai Men Dong (*Tuber Ophiopogonis Japonici*) 1/2 portion
- Bai Fu Ling (*Sclerotium Poriae Cocos*) 1/2 portion
- White honey 5 portions

Mix all ingredients together, then cook on a low boil for several hours until it becomes thickened. Take 1 teaspoon per day with warm wine.

Forever Young (Rong Yang Bu Lao Fang)
Source: *Miraculous Formulas (Qi Xiao Liong Fong)*

The ancient Chinese wrote poems about (and to) this formula, such is its power to prevent wrinkles and rejuvenate the face. Instead of nourishing the kidney and liver, which is the usual herbal beauty pathway, this formula concentrates on harmonizing the entire body to facilitate abundant qi and blood flow. Ingredients:

- Shen Jiang (*Rhizoma Zingiberis Officinalis Recens*) 200 g
- Da Zao (*Fructus Zizyphi Jujubae*) 100 g
- Salt 15 g
- Gan Cao (*Radix Glycyrrhizae Uralensis*) 30 g
- Ding Xiang (*Flos Caryophylli*) 5 g
- Chen Xiang (*Lignum Aquilariae*) 5 g
- Huo Xiang (*Herba Agastaches seu Pogostemi*) 40 g

Mix all the ingredients together, blend into powder, and keep in cool, dry place. Take 10 grams each day with warm water.

Eight Treasures (Ba Zhen Tang)
Source: *Catalogued Essentials for Correcting the Body* (*Zheng Ti Lei Yao*)

This is one of the most famous traditional Chinese herbal formulas. Its usage is wide and varied, and includes facial beauty concerns such as pale and lust less complexion, puffiness of eyes, and thin, shallow wrinkles due to qi and blood deficiency. Ingredients:

- Ren Shen (*Radix Ginseng*)
- Bai Zhu (*Rhizoma Atractylodis Macrocephalae*)
- Bai Fu Ling (*Sclerotium Poriae Cocos*)
- Dang Gui (*Radix Angelicae Sinensis*)
- Chuan Xiong (*Radix Ligustici Chuanxiong*)
- Bai Shao (*Radix Paeoniae Lactiflorae*)
- Shu Di Huang (*Radix Rehmanniae Glutinosae*)
- Zhi Gan Cao (*Radix Glycyrrhizae Uralensis*) (Honey Fried Licorice)

Two Chinese dates and 3 thin slices of fresh ginger are usually added to this formula. Use ready-made pill form.

Six Rehmannia (Liu Wei Di Huang Wan)
Source: *Collections of Treatment for Children's Disease* (*Xiao Er Yao Zheng Zhi Jue*)

This is a classic formula for treating kidney yin deficiency conditions. It can be used for facial rejuvenations concerns such as dark eye circles, age spots and facial discolorations due to kidney deficiency. Ingredients:

- Shu Di Huang (*Radix Rehmanniae Glutionsae Conquitae*)

- Shan Yao (*Radix Dioscoreae Oppositae*)
- Shan Zhu Yu (*Fructus Corni Officinalis*)
- Ze Xie (*Rhizoma Alismatis Orientalis*)
- Fu Ling (*Sclerotium Poriae Cocos*)
- Mu Dan Pi (*Cortex Moutan Radicis*)

Use ready-made pill form.

Tonify Middle and Fortify Qi Formula (Bu Zhong Yi Qi Tan)
Source: *Discussion of the Spleen and Stomach* (*Pi Wei Lun*)

A classic formula used for tonifying qi and middle jao, strengthens digestive system. It can be used for sagging of face and puffiness of eyes due to qi deficiency. Ingredients:

- Huang Qi (*Radix Astragali Membranacei*)
- Gan Cao (*Radix Glycyrrhizae Uralensis*)
- Ren Shen (*Radix Ginseng*)
- Dang Gui (*Radix Angelicae Sinensis*)
- Chen Pi (*Pericarpium Citri Sarcodactylis*)
- Sheng Ma (*Cimicifugae Rhizoma*)
- Chai Hu (*Bupleuri Radix*)
- Bai Zhu (*Rhizoma Atractylodis Macrocephalae*)

Use ready-to-use pill form.

Fourteen-Herb Fortifying Formula (Shi Si Wei Jiang Zhong Tang)
Source: *Tai Ping's Various Formulas* (*Tai Ping Sheng Hui Fang*)

This particular formula tonifies qi and blood, harmonizes ying and wei, promotes radiant complexion, and treats facial discolorations due to disharmony of ying and wei causing chronic deficient conditions. Ingredients:

- Bai Zhu (*Rhizoma Atractylodis Macrocephalae*)
- Bai Shao (*Radix Paeoniae Lactiflorae*)
- Dang Gui (*Radix Angelicae Sinensis*)
- Zhi Gan Cao (*Radix Glycyrrhizae Uralensis*) (Honey Fried Licorice)
- Ren Shen (*Radix Ginseng*)
- Mai Men Dong (*Tuber Ophiopogonis Japonici*)
- Chuan Xiong (*Radix Ligustici Chuanxiong*)
- Rou Gui (*Cortex Cinnamomi Cassiae*)
- Fu Zi (*Radix Lateralis Aconiti Carmichaeli Praeparata*)
- Rou Cong Rong (*Cistanches Deserticolae*)
- Ban Xia (*Rhizoma Pinelliae Ternatae*)
- Huang Qi (*Radix Astragali Membranacei*)
- Fu Ling (*Sclerotium Poriae Cocos*)
- Shu Di Huang (*Radix Rehmanniae Glutionsae Conquitae*)

Take the same amount of all the ingredients, mix, and blend into fine powder. Take 15 grams per day with warm water.

Anti-aging Facial Nourishing Formula (Que Lao Yang Zhong Wan)
Source: *Tai Ping's Various Formulas* (*Tai Ping Sheng Hui Fang*)

This simple formula nourishes qi and yin at the same time, reverses the aging process of the face, and treats facial wrinkles. Ingredients:

- Fresh juice of Huang Jing (*Rhizoma Polygonati*)

- Fresh juice of Sheng Di Huang (*Radix Rehmanniae Glutionsae*)
- Honey

Mix 3 portions of fresh Huang Jing juice with 1 portion of fresh Sheng Di Huang juice. Add 2 portions of honey. Mix all of the ingredients together. Place on a low boil until thick and sticky. Cool and roll into small balls (about the size of pennies). Taking one ball per day with warm wine, three times pcr day.

Chapter 9
Topical Herbal Formulas for Facial Rejuvenation

Over thousands of years practice, TCM has accumulated hundreds of external-use formulas for different skin conditions, which includes topical applications for facial rejuvenation. Unfortunately, there is no Chinese medical book that contains all the formulas; they are scattered in different books from different authors and from different dynasties. For the purpose of this book, some easily prepared formulas are introduced here:

Seven White Cream (Qi Bai Fang)
Source: *Medical Formulas from the Palace Hospital* (*Yu Yuan Yao Fang*)

This cream can be used for regular skin care, especially for age/dark spots and facial discolorations, brightening the skin, and dry skin conditions. It treats rough skin, facial discolorations, and wrinkles. Ingredients:

- Bai Zhi (*Radix Angelicae Dahuricae*) 30 g
- Bai Lian (*Radix Ampelopsis*) 30 g
- Bai Zhu (*Rhizoma Atractylodis Macrocephalae*) 30 g
- Bai Ji (*Rhizoma Bletilla Striatae*) 15 g
- Bai Fu Ling (*Sclerotium Poriae Cocos*) 9 g
- Bai Fu Zhi (*Rhizoma Typhonii Gigantei*) 9 g

- Xi Xin (*Herba cum Radice Asari*) 9 g

Preparation: Clean the above herbs, then blend them together into a fine powder. Mix the powder with egg white to form a thick paste and make into small balls. Sun dry the herbal ball.

Usage: Each night after washing the face, take a small ball and dissolve it in a small container of warm water. Apply the solution to the face.

Princess Yong He Herbal Facial Wash (Yong He Gu Zu Xi Mian Yao)
Source: *Tai Ping's Various Formulas (Tai Ping Sheng Hui Fang)*

This formula expels wind, promotes blood flow, and nourishes and beautifies the face. It is used for dull complexion and wrinkly skin. Ingredients:

- Ji Gu Xiong (*Radix Crotonis Crassifoli*) 90g
- Zao Jiao (*Fructus Gleditsiae Sinensis*) 300g
- Bai Zhi (*Radix Angelicae Dahuricae*) 150g
- Gua Lou Ren (Semen Trichosanthis) 150g
- Chuan Xiong (*Radix Ligustici Chuanxiong*) 150g
- Soybean 250g
- Chi Xiao Dou (*Semen Phaseoli Calcarati*) 250g

Preparation: Roast Zao Jiao first, then take out the peel. Mix all the ingredients together, blend into a very fine powder. Keep in a tight jar.

Usage: Take 1 teaspoonful of the powder and mix with 1 ounce of warm water. Use as a facial wash mornings and evenings.

Chapter 10
Ping Zhang's Nefeli Internal and Topical Herbal Formulas
for Facial Rejuvenation

As a practitioner of Traditional Chinese Medicine, I believe what the Chinese sages professed—that beauty has to come from inside. TCM identifies many individual herbs as treating individual facial concerns, as well as many effective ancient anti-aging formulas for facial beauty. However, with respect to the formulas, especially internal formulas, it is not very clear from the literature which ones treat which concerns. For example, no formula is specially identified for treating wrinkles or dark circles.

Through many years of training and practice, I have been able to adapt the ancient formulas in such a way as to arrive at specific formulas for specific facial concerns. These formulas, totally based on TCM, encompass the same basic herbal knowledge known and used for thousands of years.

My line of facial rejuvenation formulas is not just dedicated to treat beauty problems. For example, if a patient suffers from seasonal allergies, it is still important to take the appropriate herbal supplement, not just for eye beauty concerns, but also for the underlying sinus condition. If, for example, a patient has general sub-health conditions, Nefeli Complete Balance may be the appropriate herbal solution, though it is only secondarily taken for facial beauty. The root problem must be treated, even though the patient's first concern may be a beautiful face.

Another example: Nefeli Healthy Hair rejuvenates the hair and helps promote hair growth. Although it might be prescribed for hair loss at the same time, the patient's face will be rejuvenated because the formula addresses the deficiency of kidney essence and liver blood that not only gave rise to the hair loss but also left the patient with a lusterless complexion.

In formulating my herbal-based skin care lines, I have found that the original ancient formulas are wonderfully effective but difficult to use today. This is because 1) the ingredients are hard to find, 2) the procedure is sometimes impossible to follow, and 3) the odor of the original formula may be difficult to accept. But because the wisdom of these formulas is so great, I persisted through trial and error to come up with this line of herbal-based skin care formulas. They have the same effectiveness as the ancient formulas yet acceptable to today's user.

Our bodies are an interconnected web. Therefore, all the formulas are designed to correct internal imbalance. For instance, a discolored face can be due to kidney yin deficiency. To correct it, the patient may need an herbal formula to treat her menopausal condition as the root treatment. A patient with eye bags and puffy eyes may have kidney yang deficiency. Not until the sinus condition is treated and the body's defense system is strengthened will her dark circles go away. To treat her condition, Nefeli Cold and Allergy Care herbal supplement would be prescribed.

With the guidance of Traditional Chinese Medicine principles, I developed my anti-aging line of supplements and skin care products that tap the underlying causes of facial concerns.

10.1 Ping's Nefeli Herbal Supplements

Nefeli Complete Balance

Design purpose of this formula:
What makes Traditional Chinese Medicine different from much Western medicine is that it stresses prevention. The goal in practicing TCM as a healing medicine is not just to let the patient settle for being "not sick"; rather they should expect to enjoy true health.

"True health" means endless physical and mental stamina. It means a finely tuned immune system that protects the body from any invading organism. It means a toxin-free internal environment. It means a stronger, more energetic person whose happiness and well-being are reflected in his or her smooth skin, clear complexion, and bright, smiling eyes. Therefore, internal balance is the true source of health.

Nefeli Complete Balance is the herbal formula to recognize that such true health can only come from realizing the two words in its name—*complete balance.*

Healing properties:
It is a basic principle of Chinese medicine that health is the natural result of achieving balance in the body's yin and yang in the five basic elements, and in the flow of the life force known as qi. Those principles are in every bottle of Nefeli Complete Balance, a daily herbal supplement that enhances the body's own tremendous healing power. If there is disease, Nefeli Complete Balance will fight it off. If there is no disease, Nefeli Complete Balance will strengthen and protect the body.

Nefeli Complete Balance also means spiritual health. Optimum health is linked with the body, mind, and soul. Western science acknowledges that stress, emotional overload, or spiritual dissatisfaction can impact our well-being. Chinese tradition recognizes that we are innately endowed with three "treasures"—essence, spirit, and energy (qi)—which work in harmony so we may function in the universe. If there is imbalance, that harmony breaks down. Nefeli Complete Balance is designed to nourish and balance the three treasures so that we may realize our whole potential and optimum health.

Health benefits and beauty facts of major herbs in this formula:

Nefeli Complete Balance consists of 14 time-honored Chinese healing herbs, carefully selected and blended to achieve ultimate synergy and maximum potency. All are rich in vitamins and antioxidants. More important, all embody ancient Chinese healing wisdom. Here are some outstanding examples of the herbs in this formula:

Ling Zhi (*Ganoderma*)
This is a superior Chinese herb that calms the mind and the spirit, strengthens heart energy, and nourishes the liver. It has been lauded by Chinese sages as a longevity herb that prevents aging and improves mental capacity and memory. It is also considered an immune system enhancer thanks to its high molecular weight in polysaccharides, triterpenes, ganoderic acids, sterols, amino acids, vitamins, coumarin, mannitol, and adenosine. Studies suggest that it may reduce allergies, lower the risk of heart disease, and inhibit tumor growth.

Chinese Ginseng
Ginseng is known as the "king" of Chinese herbs. It fights fatigue and stress by tonifying all the body's internal organ systems as it increases blood and oxygen supply to the brain. It protects the liver, improves general metabolism, strengthens the immune system, and anchors soul and spirit.

It promotes longevity and endurance. Modern studies suggest it benefits the heart system. Ginseng contains panaxatriol; 17 amino acids; vitamins A, E, B2, and niacin; and more than 20 different minerals.

Hong Jing Tain (*Rhodiola*)
This powerful Tibetan medicine is famous for its strong antitoxic properties.
- It is widely known for its anti-aging and beautifying powers.
- It greatly shortens recovery time from illness.
- It increases the attention span and sharpens the memory.
- It is loaded with antitoxicity and free-radical-fighting ingredients, including salidrosides, rhodosin, tyrosol, dendrolasin, safranal, 17 essential amino acids, 21 trace elements, vitamins, volatile oils, alkaloid, and flavones.

Nefeli Complete Balance is suggested as supplement for individuals looking for a superior daily herbal "vitamin" to maintain and improve overall health and well-being. It is also recommended for those with the following concerns:
- Stress, fatigue, or shortness of breath
- Irritability
- Panic attacks
- Memory and thinking power
- Insomnia, dream-disturbed sleep, night sweats
- Low will power or spirit
- Constipation, indigestion, slow metabolism
- Immune deficiency, allergies, or frequent colds
- Signs of aging, such as dull complexion, tired eyes, and sagging facial muscles

Nefeli Brighten Complexion

Design purpose of this formula:
Healthy, clear, and bright skin is an important concern when considering our facial beauty. Nefeli Brighten Complexion provides an alternative noninvasive solution for resolving facial discolorations, including age spots and dark pigmentations. It treats the root of the problem. Obviously, overexposure to the sun can be very damaging to the skin. However, other factors contributing to discolorations may be hormonal imbalance, skin disease, medications, and aging in general. According to TCM theory, these disharmonies of the skin are mainly related to the improper balance of the liver, kidney, and spleen.

Based on these principles, Nefeli Brighten Complexion is formulated as a "root" treatment to regulate and harmonize the liver, kidney and spleen function, while additional selected herbs have been included to help brighten the face.

Healing properties:
Herbs in this formula are selected based on their special properties, documented in China's most famous herbal texts. This formula supports and cleanses the body, while helping to improve the condition of dull complexion, dark spots, and other discolorations.

Health benefits and beauty facts of major herbs in this formula:

Dong Gua Ren (*Semen Benincasae Hispidae*)
- Nourishes the lungs, reduces water swellings, tonifies the liver.

- Enlightens the body, clears dark spots and brightens the face
- Contains saponins, urea, and guanidine.

Bai Zhi (*Radix Angelicae Dahuricae*)
- Reduces swelling, drains pus, promotes healing of skin
- Fragrances the body
- Clears wind and itch from the face
- Clears facial discolorations and dark spots
- nourishes the face
- Contains vaporizing oil, atractylol, atractylon, vitamin A, selina-4,ien-8-one, attractylenolide, 8-b-ethoxy atractylenolide III

Fu Ling (*Sclerotium Poriae Cocos*)
- Improves digestive functioning
- Drains the system of unwanted fluids
- Calms the spirit
- Improves a lusterless complexion
- Relieves discolorations and dark spots
- Contains many organic acids such as pachymose, albuninoid, fiber, pachymaran, β-pachyman, β-pachymanase, pachymic acid, tumulosic acid, eburioic acid, pinicolic acid, poricoic, and fatty acids such as caprylic acid, undecanoic acid, lauric acid, dodecenole acid, and palmitic acid. It also contains ergosterol, gum, histadine, chline, chitin, protein, fats, glucose, sterols, histamines, lecithin, lipase, choline, adenine, as well traces minerals.

Sheng Di Huang (*Radix Rehmanniae Glutinosae*)
- Cools and nourishes blood
- Provides the ability to center the spirit

- Tonifies kidney water and true yin, thus providing relief for dry skin
- Nourish the skin and beautifies the face
- Replenishes bone marrow
- Elongates life
- Contains beta-stitoserol, mannitol, stigmasterol, campesterol, rehmannia, catapol, arginine, and glucose

Gou Qi Zi (*Fructus Lycii*)
- Strengthens ligaments and bones
- Enlightens the body
- Delays the aging process
- Tonifies insufficient essence and qi
- Beautifies and brightens the skin tone
- Benefits the eyes
- Promotes longevity
- Contains betain, zeaxanthin, physalein, beta-carotene, thiamine, riboflavin, vitamin C, B1, B2, B-sitosterol (an anti-inflammatory agent), linoleic acid (a fatty acid), immunological active polysaccharides, sesquiterpenoids, and trace minerals.

Nefeli Brighten Complexion is recommended for people with the following concerns:
- Age spots
- Facial discolorations due to hormonal imbalance and other undifferentiated pathologies
- Brown spots due to sun exposure

Nefeli Wrinkle Smoother

Design purpose of this formula:
Facelifts, light treatments, Botox, and other injections are currently being used to lessen the appearance of wrinkles.

TCM offers an alternative holistic, noninvasive treatment for wrinkle care. Wrinkles are a result of the natural aging process that begins after the age of 25. However, through TCM care, wrinkle formation can be delayed, reducing it to an unrecognizable level.

Healing properties:
Herbs in this formula are selected based on their special properties, documented in China's most famous herbal texts. This formula helps nourish the body from within to prevent signs of aging, while smoothing wrinkles and diminishing the appearance of fine lines.

Health benefits and beauty facts of major herbs used in this formula:

E Jiao (*Gelatinum Corii Asini*)
This particular herb is processed from the skin of a donkey. It contains a type of protein that, when hydrolyzed, releases gelatinized amino acids that are easily absorbed by our digestive system. E Jiao thus tonifies the blood, balances the level of calcium, and improves nutrient supply to the body.

For centuries, it has been used as the major herb for wrinkled conditions of the skin. E Jiao is a blood tonic and is widely used to stop bleeding, nourish yin, and moisten dryness. E Jiao retards the aging process, moistens and replenishes dry skin, diminishes wrinkles, and beautifies skin tone.

It contains collagen hydrolyzed into amino acids: including lysine, arginine, histamine, cysteine, tryptophan, hydroxyproline, serine, aspartic acid, threonine, glutamic acid, praline, glycine, alanine, valine, methionine, isoleucine, leucine, tyrosine, and phenylalanine.

Ginseng (*Radix Ginseng*)

As one of the most precious Chinese medicines, this superior herb is considered to be the "king" of Chinese herbs. Its ancient name is "Magic Returning to Wrinkled Face." Ginseng takes six to seven years to harvest, the best varieties growing wild in the northern and eastern mountain regions of China and Korea.

Ginseng's benefits are great in number as have mentioned in this book before. Of major significance is its ability to tonify and nourish the heart, lungs, spleen, kidneys, and liver organ systems; calm the spirit; benefit the eyes; and enhance intelligence. Long-term usage of ginseng can increase longevity, enlighten the body, and improve the body's total well-being.

Modern research shows ginseng plays an important part in the prevention of wrinkle formation. Its main ingredients, panaxatriol, 17 amino acids, vitamins A, E, B2, niacin, and more than 20 different kinds of minerals, are essential for maintaining healthy and beautiful skin.

Dang Gui (*Radix Angelicae Sinensis*)

The Chinese term *dang gui* refers to a wife who misses her faraway husband and prays that he will come back soon. Dang Gui is the most important Chinese herb used for gynecological conditions. Its function works uniquely by harmonizing and moving blood. According to the ancient herbal texts, Dang Gui treats almost all conditions related to gynecology, while at the same time beautifies the skin by improving blood circulation.

Dang Gui cleans the "garbage" from the skin and brightens the face as it nourishes and replenishes the nutrients to the skin. It is, therefore, an important herb for the beautification of the skin and the prevention and treatment of wrinkles.

Modern scientific research shows dang gui contains major ingredients that contribute to healthy skin, including succinic acid, nicotinic acid, uracil, adenine, butylidene phthalide, biotin, polysaccharide, carotene, B-sitosterol, Ferulic acid (a strong antioxidant), 19 amino acids (which serve the function of helping tighten the skin and diminish wrinkles), vitamins A, E, B12, and trace minerals.

Research has also shown that Dang Gui can improve blood circulation, protect the liver, resist vitamin E deficiency, and increase whole body metabolism. Dang Gui's antibiotic effect and antioxidant property (ability to clear free radicals, the major factor in wrinkle formation) make it an invaluable herb in this formula.

Traditionally, this herb belongs to the category of blood tonics. Accordingly, it has the properties to tonify and invigorate blood, regulate menses, alleviate PMS pain, moisten the intestines and unblock constipation, as well as retard aging and diminish wrinkles.

Huang Jing (*Rhizoma Polygonati*)

This herb is said to make the face "as beautiful and young as a young child." Huang Jing's properties have a calming effect upon the five internal organs. Long-term usage can enlighten the body, elongate life, help tendons and bones, benefit digestion, and nourish the heart and lungs. Huang jing contains azetidine-2-carboxylic acid, aspartic acid, homoserine, diamin butyric acid, digitalis glycoside and eleven different kinds of amino acids.

Modern scientific research down in china on this herb finds that Huang Jing may increase the immune function of the human cell, increase the T-cell percentages in the body, improve conditions of anemia, improve digestive functioning, and increase libido. At the same time, Huang Jing can help delay the aging process of internal organs and skin, and reduce facial discolorations due to aging.

Nefeli Wrinkle Smoother is recommended for people who wish to:
- Prevent wrinkles due to aging and premature aging
- Diminish wrinkles due to external environmental factors such as sun and wind exposure
- Diminish wrinkles due to unhealthy living styles and conditions
- Diminish wrinkles due to deficient body conditions
- Try a natural, alternative way for healing body conditions

Nefeli Eye Refresh

Design purpose of this formula:
For over 2000 years, TCM has accumulated rich and refined treatments for the total eye system. It has provided thousands of valuable methods, including herbal therapy and acupuncture, to treat eye problems in an effective and natural way.

Nefeli Eye Refresh formula works for the total care of the eyes by enhancing healthy general body function, while, at the same time, directly taking care of local concerns.

Healing properties:
According to the sages, the eye is the place where essence and qi from our internal organs pull together. It is the window that represents our spiritual vitality. It is the opening of the liver and the representative of the heart. The beauty and health of the eyes are directly related to these organ functions.

Herbs in this formula are traditionally used in China to help improve vision, diminish dark circles, and smooth puffiness around the eyes.

Health benefits and beauty facts of major herbs used in this formula:

Huang Qi (Radix Astragali Membranacei)
According to Chinese literature on herbal medicine, this superior herb tonifies qi and blood, strengthens and increases spleen and stomach qi, stabilizes the body's surface, promotes urination, and reduces swelling.

Because of these functions, Huang Qi is included in this formula to strengthen the body and help reduce eye bags and puffiness around the eyes.

Huang Qi contains activants of coumarin and flavonoid derivatives, which have the function of anti-free-radical activity, and saponins, which benefits the immune system. Huang Qi also contains polysaccharides, which have anti-rhinoviral activity. In addition, it contains 21 amino acids and 14 minerals.

Gou Qi Zi (*Fructus Lycii*)
For centuries, Chinese medical literature has considered this herb to be a superior treasure for the health of the eyes. According to the literature, this herb nourishes liver and kidney function, replenishes vital essence, delays the aging process, and brightens the eyes. Gou Qi Zi contains betain, zeaxanthin, physalein, beta-carotene, thiamine, riboflavin, immunologically active polysaccharides, sesquiterpenoids, and trace minerals.

Chuan Xiong (*Radix Ligustici Chuanxiong*)
This herb, considered a superior herb according to Chinese herbal texts, invigorates the blood, promotes the movement of qi, and expels wind, especially from the face. It is an

excellent herb to help relieve dark circles around the eyes and eye bags. Chuang Xiong contains tetramethylpyrazine, perlilyrine, ferulic acid, chrysopganol, sedanoic acid, 4-hycoxy-3-butyphthalide.

Tu Si Zi (*Semen Cuscutae Chinensis*)

This superior yang tonic nourishes deficiencies in the body. Tu Si Zi promotes overall energy, replenishes the body's vital essence, benefits bone marrow, tonifies liver and kidney essence, and benefits spleen and kidney function. If taken long-term, Tu Si Zi has the ability to brighten the eyes, enlighten the body, and elongate life. Tu Si Zi contains vitamin A, glycosides, cholesterol, campestetol, and B-sitosterol.

Mu Zei (*Herba Equiseti Hiemalis*)

Mu Zei is a major Chinese herb used to treat eye disorders. It has a special ability to clear superficial visual obstructions such as painful swelling, cloudy or blurred vision, and excessive tearing due to wind-heat obstructing the eyes. It contains palustrine, dimethylsulfone, ferulic and caffeic acid, vanillin, thymine, and aconitic acid.

This formula is recommended for people who suffer from the following concerns:
- Environmental factors
- Aging
- Stress
- Deficient body conditions
- Blurred vision, red and swollen eyes, or cloudy vision
- Dark eye circles
- Puffy eyes

Nefeli Healthy Hair

Design purpose of this formula:
Millions of people suffer from hair loss. Hair not only serves as a crown on the top of the head, but as a protection for the scalp. Having healthy, beautiful, full hair is a symbol of health and youth. Its presence supports our spiritual and physical health.

TCM and proper nutrition offer effective treatment for hair loss and hair rejuvenation.

According to traditional theory, hair is considered a surplus of blood. The liver stores blood, and the kidney stores essence. The healthy abundance of liver and kidney essences is reflected in the health and beauty of our hair.

Nefeli Healthy Hair uses this guideline to meet the needs of those with dry, broken, and damaged hair. It is exceptionally effective for men and women suffering from hair loss.

Healing properties:
Herbs in this formula are traditionally used in China to nourish and balance the body's internal system to help prevent hair loss and promote hair growth.

This specially designed formula helps to nourish hair, stop hair loss, and promote hair growth in the following ways:
- Tonifies liver and kidneys
- Promotes blood, energy circulation to the scalp
- Detoxifies and cleans grease and dampness on the scalp to maintain clean conditions for hair follicles

Health benefits and beauty facts of major herbs used in this formula:

He Shou Wu (*Radix Polygoni Multiflori*)
He Shou Wu has the healing ability to nourish qi and blood. It replenishes the essences of liver and kidney, and protects the heart. The use of He Shou Wu is vital to the treatment of graying hair and for the beautification of the face. Taken long-term, this herb can also strengthen tendons and bones, benefit essence and marrow, and promote anti-aging and longevity.

He Shou Wu contains lecithin, which plays an important role in blocking cholesterol uptake from the plasma into the liver. In this manner, he shou wu can prevent the deposition of cholesterol into places in the arterial wall. Its strong anti-aging function works by increasing SOD (Superoxide Dismutase) activity in different organ systems.

Shu Di Huang (*Radix Rehmanniae Glutinosae Conquitae*)
This is another valuable herb that tonifies blood and replenishes the vitality of the kidney and liver essences, so very relevant for healthy hair growth. Shu Di Huang nourishes the hair, helping to retard hair loss and premature graying.

Modern research suggests that this herb contains 15 amino acids and more than 29 trace minerals, which provide nutrients to the roots of the hair, making it stable for growth.

According to modern research, Shu Di Huang also has antibacterial and anti-inflammatory properties that benefit hair growth by cleaning and calming the skin.

Ce Bai Ye (*Cacumen Biotae Orientalis*)
This herb nourishes source qi and internal organs. It strengthens the body to fight aging, cools the blood, stops hair loss due to heat in the blood, and prevents premature graying of hair.

According to modern research, Ce Bai Ye has an antibiotic effect and is known to be very effective for alopecia. It contains volatile oil, flavonoids, quercitrin, tannin, vitamin C, and isopimaric acid.

Ju Hua (*Flos Chrysanthemi Morifolii*)
Ju Hua is an excellent herb to clear heat, expel wind, detoxify the body, promote hair growth, and treat premature graying of hair. Ju Hua works as a guiding herb and helps to bring the rest of the formula to the face and head. Ju Hua contains alkaloids, volatile oil, sesquiterpene lactones, flavonoids, adenine, chorine, stachydrine, chrysanthemum, and vitamin B1.

Nefeli Healthy Hair is recommended for people who suffer from the following conditions:
- Hair loss and/or premature graying of hair
- Sub-health conditions due to overwork of the brain, stress, insufficient sleep, or irregular lifestyle
- Side effects of medications; chemotherapy
- Side effects of poor quality hair care products
- Failure of other products to work

Nefeli Weight Management

Design purpose of this formula:
Being overweight not only affects how we look but also is considered by almost all cultures to be a condition of imbalance posing serious consequences to health. Highly processed and "fast" foods, compounded by highly stressed

lifestyles, often leave us overweight and at great risk for disease. For centuries, the Chinese people have recognized that being overweight is an unhealthy condition. Nefeli brings to you this unique weight management formula in the pursuit of health, balance, and longevity.

Healing properties:
In this multidimensional formula, Chinese botanicals are traditionally used to help strengthen and promote the body's metabolism, cleanse toxic buildups, maintain optimum condition, and keep the body healthy and fit. This formula treats weight problems in the following ways:

- Increases the body's metabolism
- Controls appetite
- Detoxifies the body

Health benefits and beauty facts of major herbs used in this formula:

Huang Qi (*Radix Astragali Membranacei*)
Huang Qi is a superior herb to tonify qi. It strengthens and raises spleen and stomach qi, stabilizes the body's surface, tonifies qi and blood, promotes urination, and reduces swelling. Huang Qi can therefore successfully be used as a primary herb to strengthen the overall body condition.

Huang Qi contains activants of coumarin and flavonoid derivatives (which clear free radicals), saponins (which benefit the immune system), and polysaccharides (which has anti-rhinoviral activity). Additionally, it contains 21 amino acids and 14 minerals.

Fu Ling (*Sclerotium Poriae Cocos*)
Fu Ling is said to leach out dampness, tonify the spleen, and calm the spirit. If taken long-term, it can nourish the spirit, reduce hunger, and delay aging.

Fu Ling contains protein, lecithin, histamines, and many trace minerals that help to increase the body's immune function.

Shan Zha (*Fructus Gardeniae Jasminoidis*)
Shan Zha is well known for its ability to reduce and clear out food stagnation, especially due to meat or greasy foods. It promotes qi movement and removes blood stasis.

Shan Zha contains crategoli acid, citric acid, tartaric acid, flavone compounds, sugars, glycosides, and vitamins C and B. Modern research has recently included Shan Zha in the treatment of hypertension and high cholesterol, making it a perfect, natural, and healthy cleanser for our bodies.

He Ye (*Folium Nelumbinis Nuciferae*)
This herb clears heat, promotes urination at the same time raises spleen yang qi, and clears heat stagnation in the lower burner.

He Ye contains nelumbino, nuciferino, and pronuciferine. Recently, it has been widely used for weight loss due to its action to suppress appetite and break down fat.

Huang Jing (*Rhizoma Polygonati*)
For centuries Huang Jing has been used to nourish the body and benefit qi, especially of the heart and lungs. It tonifies spleen and stomach qi and yin, as well as kidney essence. Therefore, it can be said to benefit and calm the five internal organs.

According to herbal testing, taking Huang Jing long-term can enlighten the body without eating grains (food), and elongate life.

This herb contains azetidine-2carboxylid acid, aspartic acid, homoserine, diaminobutyric acid, digitalis glycoside, and 11 amino acids.

Modern medical research finds that it can increase the immune function of the human cell, increase T-cell percentages in the body, and delay the aging process for internal organs and skin. Additionally, Huang Jing improves conditions of anemia, prevents hardening of blood vessels, and improves digestive functioning.

Nefeli Weight Management is recommended for overweight people with the following concerns:
- Excessive appetite
- Low energy
- Low metabolism
- High cholesterol
- Constipation

Nefeli Menopause Soother

Design purpose of this formula:
With most of the baby boomer generation entering mid-life, many women are now suffering from the uncomfortable symptoms of premenopause and menopause. Breast cancer, heart disease, blood clots, and stroke have recently been linked to hormonal replacement therapy.

TCM has successfully been treating menopausal conditions since ancient times. It serves as a natural and wonderful substitute for hormone replacement.

Healing properties:
According to the *Yellow Emperor's Inner Classic,* women at about the age of 49 are deprived of kidney qi. Blood and essence become insufficient. These deficiencies can cause disturbing and, at times, alarming signs and symptoms referred to as "menopausal syndrome." To improve the

symptoms associated with menopausal syndrome, I developed this formula based on years of experience and according to TCM healing theories. It helps the body to nourish the kidney in particular, including yin, yang, and essence.

Specially selected herbs in this formula are traditionally used in China to address the underlying condition of menopause. This formula further helps to relieve the signs and symptoms of menopause, such as hot flashes, fatigue, insomnia, day and night sweats, mood wings, anxiety, dizziness, vaginal dryness, dry mouth and skin, decreased vision and hearing, and memory loss.

Health benefits and beauty facts of major herbs used in this formula:

Sheng Di Huang (*Radix Rehmanniae Glutinosae*)
According to traditional Chinese herbal texts, when used fresh, sheng di huang cools the blood, nourishes yin, generates fluids, tonifies the five internal organs, replenishes bone marrow, and nourishes and benefits the skin. When used prepared (cooked), sheng di huang tonifies the blood. Sheng Di Huang is highly effective in the treatment of hot flashes, dizziness, night sweats, and dry and wrinkled skin due to blood and yin deficiency.

Sheng Di Huang contains polysaccharides, 15 amino acids (which help to nourish and tighten the skin), and more than 29 trace minerals that provide nutrients to the skin and vitamin A (an anti-wrinkle agent). Sheng Di Huang also has antibacterial and anti-inflammatory properties, which play an important role in calming the skin to make it stable. This herb is very effective for anti-aging, skin rashes, and rough and wrinkled skin.

The prepared form of this herb is called Shou Di Huang. It has a slightly warm property and functions more to tonify the liver and kidney, tonify the blood, beautify the skin, and prevent and smooth wrinkles.

Xian Ling Pi (*Herba Epimedii*)
This herb is known to tonify both kidney yin and yang. It benefits energy, strengthens tendons and bones, improves memory, and alleviates joint pain. Xian Ling Pi has the ability to regulate the menses, address frequent urination, and raise low libido. Xian Ling Pi contains flavone compounds, fat, saponins, and essential oil.

Nefeli Menopause Soother is recommended for premenopausal and menopausal women with the following concerns:

- Irritability
- Fatigue
- Insomnia
- Memory loss
- Anxiety
- Hot flashes and/or sweats
- Night sweats
- Dry mouth and skin
- Decreased vision and hearing
- Vaginal dryness and irritation
- Wrinkles
- Mood swings

Nefeli Herbal Passion

Design purpose of this formula:
People have always understood the importance of having enough sexual energy in their lives. A healthy balanced state of desire and performance helps to relieve tension and stress, improve sleep, benefit relationships, increase self-confidence, and delay the aging process.

For centuries, people have searched for better ways of promoting and increasing a happier and healthier sex life. TCM provides an effective way to take care of these concerns. According to the classics, low sexuality is the result of a kidney qi and essence deficiency that has been brought about in various ways.

Nefeli Herbal Passion formula aspires to replenish kidney essence, promote blood flow, and rejuvenate the fire of life's gate (Ming Men). It helps to support the body's overall physiological function. Nefeli Herbal Passion regenerates the body's energy, increasing endurance and the body's ability to handle stress and fatigue.

Healing properties of this formula:
This balanced formula of specially selected Chinese herbs have been used for hundreds of years to replenish the vital essences of both kidney yin and yang, tonify qi and blood, and promote blood circulation. Nefeli Herbal Passion produces superior internal body balance with increased stamina and sense of well being, for both men and women.

Health benefits and beauty facts of major herbs used in this formula:

Xian Ling Pi (*Herba Epimedii*)
This herb tonifies kidney yin and yang, benefits energy, strengthens tendons and bones, improves memory, relieves joint pain, and regulates the menses.

According to modern research, this herb stimulates the sensory nerves to directly increase sexual desire, for men and women. It also increases sperm production.

Xian Ling Pi contains flavone compounds, fat, saponins, and essential oil.

Tu Si Zi (*Semen Cuscutae Chinensis*)
This superior herb replenishes liver and kidney yin and yang, tonifies and secures the body's vital essences for the symptoms of impotence, nocturnal emission, and premature ejaculation in men. It promotes secretion of sperm and increases sexual function.

In women, Tu Si Zi is well known to increase libido, lubricate vaginal dryness, and stabilize excessive vaginal discharge.

This herb contains vitamin A, glycosides, cholesterol, campestetol, B-sitosterol.

Jiu Zi (*Semen Allii Tuberosi*)
This herb/vegetable warms the kidneys, tonifies yang, and secures the essence. When combined with other yang tonics, Jiu Zi can strongly increase sexual drive in both men and women. Jiu Zi contains organic alkaline and Zhao Gan.

Nefeli Herbal Passion is recommended for men and women with the following concerns:
- Women experiencing decreased sexual drive, vaginal discharges, low energy, sore back or legs
- Men experiencing impotence, low sexual energy, low energy, spermatorrhea, nocturnal emission

Nefeli Cold and Allergy Care

Design purpose of this formula:
Each year, millions of dollars are spent for the symptomatic relief of seasonal allergies and sinus cold conditions. Treating these conditions symptomatically does provide minimal relief but, unfortunately, weakens the immune system, leaving one at risk for further allergies and future cold attacks.

Traditional Chinese Medicine has an herbal answer to this problem. Nefeli Cold and Allergy Care not only relieves uncomfortable symptoms, but provides natural care for sinus-cold and allergy sufferers by fortifying the body's immune system, enabling it to fight these conditions on its own.

Healing properties:
This formula addresses sinus-cold and allergic conditions in the following ways:
- Strengthens the immune system
- Adjusts and harmonizes the yin and wei level (energy and blood level), creating a balanced condition that allows the body to gain enough strength to fight external influences
- Expels wind, clears the heat or cold, relieves external conditions

Working together, the herbs in this formula strengthen and stimulate the body's own ability to fight sinus colds, flus and seasonal allergies, while at the same time relieve the signs and symptoms associated with it.

Health benefits and beauty facts of major herbs used in this formula:

Ban Lan Gen (*Radix Isatidis seu Baphicacanthi*)
This herb clears heat, detoxifies the body, and acts as an antiviral agent. It also has strong antimicrobial and antiparasitic effects.

Jin Yin Hua (*Flos Lonicerae Japonicae*) and **Lian Qiao** (*Fructus Forsythiae Suspensae*)
These herbs clear heat and relieve toxicity. Jin Yin Hua has an antiviral and anti-infectious effect. Lian Qiao has an antimicrobial and antiparasitic effect.

Xin Yi Hua (*Flos Magnoliae*) and **Chang Er Zi** (*Fructus Xanthii Sibirici*)

These herbs work together to open the nasal passage and relieve allergy symptoms. Xin Yi Hua has effect on the nasal mucosa. Chang Er Zi has anantimicrobial effect.

Da Zao (*Fructus Zizyphi Jujubae*) and **Bai Shao** (*Radix Paeoniae Lactiflorae*)

These herbs harmonize the yin and wei level to secure and strengthen the body's ability to fight external environmental attacks.

Nefeli Cold and Sinus Care is recommended for the following:
- Sinus cold and allergic conditions
- Dark eye circles and puffiness of eyes due to a sinus condition

10.2 Nefeli Topical Herbal Skin Care
Facial Rejuvenation

TCM herbal medicine for topical application has been an important part of herbal medicine treatment modality. For topical treatments, herbal formula can be taken in many different forms. For example, a dried herbal powder form can be applied to a certain area for certain internal conditions. An herbal decoction in a bath may be best for certain skin conditions and arthritic pain. An herbal ointment or liniment can be applied topically for traumatic injuries and bruises. An herbal soak or wash can be used for skin rejuvenation. There are hundreds of herbal formulas for different skin concerns.

Over the decade of my practice, I have taken steps toward skin care by making teas, oil-based applications, and masks for my patients. Through my experience I have seen that ancient skin care formulas bring great harmonizing results. However, the original herbal ingredients from ancient formulas sometimes are either hard to find or may not be acceptable, for instance, because of an unpleasant smell. In addition, the procedures to make these creams and washes can be very time-consuming or even impossible to produce. Patients demand a formula that is natural, safe, herbal-based, convenient, and nonfragrant. These requests have inspired me to do considerable research to develop effective herbal formulas for my skin products that are safe, natural, and pure. Despite some challenges, my herbal skin care line has been born. After years of trial use and further refinement, safe, pure, and effective formulas have evolved. They are all paraben free, mineral-oil free, and consist of no artificial fragrances or colors.

My skin care line serves as a basic supporting system for my facial acupuncture treatment. The line has five basic categories of skin care products, including one all-purpose skin wash:

- **All-Purpose Skin Wash**—initiates the skin healing process while cleansing the face.
- **Aged Skin/Wrinkle Care**—for wrinkles and aged skin concerns. It is designed for all skin types.

- **Bright Complexion**—releases discolorations of face, age spots, and dark spots. It promotes facial glow. It is designed for all skin types.
- **Rescue Remedies**—for emergency conditions that need the skin to be in the beat condition with instant rejuvenation result.
- **All-in-One Eye Care**—all-in-one herbal eye care designed for treating dark eye circles, eye bags, and wrinkles around eyes.
- **Cellulite Reduction**—for helping reduce cellulite and firm uneven skin tone.

These categories represent specific herbal skin care formulas, which are described below:

All-Purpose Skin Wash

- **Skin Brightening Facial Wash**—*Where skin care begins*

This all-purpose facial wash cleans and purifies the skin with a combination of herbal extracts from aloe, ginkgo biloba, and papaya, leaving the skin feeling refreshed and healthy. This wash can be used with all Nefeli skin care lines.

1. Aged Skin/Wrinkle Care—*For firming, repairing, lifting, and smoothing wrinkles*

Traditional Chinese Daoism has long offered a healing approach to facial wrinkling. Nefeli brings you that wisdom. The secret lies in powerful herbs that help you overcome the roughness and sagging that lead to fine lines and deep wrinkles. Nefeli's anti-wrinkle formulas combine traditional Chinese healing power with more recently recognized natural plant components, such as antioxidants that neutralize skin-cell-damaging free radicals. The special herbs that are used are precisely blended so they can work synergistically to fight aging. They also fight the wrinkles that go with aging by helping to re-energize and replenish of the skin at the cellular level. Such herbs are found in each of the following Nefeli anti-wrinkle formulas for smooth, supple facial skin and a stress-free face that radiates natural beauty.

- **Nefeli Intensive Wrinkle Care Mask**
  This holistic skin care herbal mask "de-stresses" the skin by using Chinese herbal extracts of astragalus root, *Angelica sinensis*, luffa, coix seed, and papaya. These potent herbs nourish, hydrate, firm, and protect the skin while diminishing the appearance of fine lines and wrinkles. The mask leaves the skin looking vibrant and young.
- **Nefeli Intensive Wrinkle Care Day Cream**
  For the first time, Nefeli uses the special legendary adaptogenic Chinese herb *Rhodiola* in its breakthrough anti-wrinkle formula. Combining ginseng, pearl, white peony root, green tea, and gingko biloba, this truly holistic Chinese herbal-based formula is as pure as it is effective in restoring youthful vigor to your skin. It nourishes, firms, energizes, and protects the skin

against environmental factors while smoothing and diminishing the appearance of fine lines and wrinkles.

- **Nefeli Intensive Wrinkle Care Night Cream**
This powerful herbal healing formula helps promote a lustrous, wrinkle-free complexion, which results from the internal harmony that is the hallmark of true skin health. Combining extracts from ganoderma, ginseng root, astragalus root, pearl, and luffa, this skin care product helps reduce the appearance of fine lines and wrinkles, nourishes and helps firm the skin, and enhances the skin's natural recovery from environmental damage.

2. Bright Complexion Care—*for promoting flawless complexion and natural skin radiance*

Chinese wisdom believes internal body disharmony, stagnation, or deficiency is the basis of much of our skin problems. Of course, external factors, such as excess sun exposure, also contribute. Nefeli's Bright Complexion formulas are designed to deal with precisely the unhealthy internal factors identified by the medical sages of ancient China. Bright Complexion formulas blend carefully selected Chinese herbs that bring a healthy balance to restore complexion to its natural brightness and evenness. The herbs also empower the skin to fight the environmental "evils" that damage complexion.

- **Nefeli Intensive Daytime Skin Brightening Cream**
Combining ancient Chinese holistic herbal healing wisdom with the latest biological and technical research

has produced this natural blend of herbal extracts from rhodiola, safflower, coix seed, pearl, and licorice. It protects the skin and helps to fight environmental factors, such as UV rays. It replenishes moisture and diminishes the appearance of dark spots and discolorations. It leaves the skin with a bright luminous complexion and naturally healthy. It is an ideal base for makeup.

- **Nefeli Intensive Nighttime Skin Brightening Cream**
  This nighttime skin brightening cream draws on ccnturics of Chinese herbal healing wisdom for flawless complexion. The natural blend of herbal extracts of pearls, poria, Chinese asparagus, atractylodis, papaya, and licorice helps activate cellular rejuvenation and promote the renewal process, diminishing the appearance of dark spots and discolorations while you sleep. This leaves the skin with a bright luminous complexion and a natural, healthy look.

3. Rescue Remedies—*for emergency skin care and dramatic results*

Sometimes looking your best can become an emergency situation. Your wedding day, high school reunion, a must-get job interview are examples of the many times when you need to look your best. Rescue Remedies is an elite set of formulas that provide instant anti-aging miracles when needed most. These products follow Traditional Chinese Medicine teachings and use time-honored Chinese herbs that work at the cellular level to bring out youth and beauty for all to see. Whether it is the eyes, face, or other skin area that needs attention, these Rescue Remedies formulas get the job done fast.

- **Nefeli Eye Rejuvenating Mask**
  This uniquely formulated multi-functional holistic eye care herbal mask uses the secrets of thousands of years of Chinese medicinal wisdom to help encourage the eye to gain natural youth and beauty from the inside out. The mask helps decrease the appearance of fine lines around eyes, dark circles, eye bags, and puffiness, leaving the eye area feeling refreshed, soothed and rejuvenated.

- **Nefeli Facial Rejuvenating Mask**
  Superior Chinese skin-healing herbs used by Chinese sages for centuries make this unique facial mask satisfy the quest to return to natural beauty. This comprehensive facial mask is a special blend that helps 1) provide time-released hydration, 2) replenish essential nutrients to the skin to prevent future signs of aging, 3) brighten and revitalize the skin's tone, 4) reduce the appearance of fine lines and wrinkles, and 5) improve elasticity of the skin. It is great for after-sun care to soothe and moisturize skin.

4. All-in-One Eye Care—*for wrinkles around the eyes, dark eye circles, and puffiness*

- **Nefeli Essential Eye Care Cream**
  Adhering strictly to the healing philosophy of Traditional Chinese Medicine, this uniquely designed

holistic eye care product is packed with ancient healing miracles whose power derives directly from nature. It delivers the healing energy of Chinese herbs to provide continuous hydration and vitality to the eye area. It reduces the appearance of fine lines, puffiness, and dark circles under or around the eyes.

5. Cellulite Reduction—*transforms phlegm accumulation, and firms the skin*

- **Nefeli Cellulite Cream**
  This unique natural cream helps to maintain the cell's natural metabolism and reduce the appearance of sagging and the uneven look of the affected area. It makes the skin feel and look natural, smoother, and firmer.

Section 4
Acupressure for Facial Rejuvenation

Chapter 11
Introduction to Acupressure Facial Rejuvenation

Acupuncture is probably the best-known, most common, and most accepted Chinese treatment method in the world today. It works for facial rejuvenation concerns. Acupressure uses the same principles as acupuncture, except pressure from the fingers or hands replaces the needles.

Over the millennia, acupressure techniques have been refined and perfected to the point that we know precisely how to apply them to treat facial beauty concerns. If you decide to give your patient needleless facial rejuvenation treatment, then the easy-to-follow acupressure protocols can be included in the treatment practice to correct those internal imbalances that are creating wrinkles, discoloration, dark circles, or eye bags, and so forth.

The Benefits of Acupressure

Like acupuncture, acupressure heals the face and body by manipulating the flow of qi in beneficial ways. It does this by activating certain energy points along the channels by means of direct pressure. Acupressure's power for facial rejuvenation works in many different ways:

- Soothes and vents the channel system
- Regulates the free flow of qi and blood
- Harmonizes yin and yang
- Encourages lymph drainage
- Facilitates nutrient absorption
- Enhances the skin's ability to "breathe"
- Promotes normal secretion from the sweat and oil glands
- Stimulates the skin's own ability for collagen production, softening the skin and smoothing wrinkles
- Regulates and stimulates internal organ system functioning
- Promotes muscle contraction

Acupressure's stimulation of the internal organs is, of course, key to its beauty benefits. By restoring organ balance, it eliminates the root cause of facial skin problems. More specifically, it promotes blood flow to the skin surface so more nutrients reach skin cells. Acupressure also has an effect on muscle contraction, reducing muscle fatigue and increasing elasticity, which in turn helps prevent sagging skin and wrinkle formation.

Acupressure and the Channels

There are typical channel systems that perform most

effectively when using acupressure routine for facial rejuvenation. The following channels are the most important for acupressure's use as a facial beauty treatment:

- **Stomach channel** (ST) – yang ming channel; full of qi and blood. When stimulating this channel, qi and blood are readily sent to the facial area.
- **Liver channel** (LIV) – also full of blood. Stimulating the liver channel purifies the blood, which helps nourish the skin.
- **Spleen channel** (SP) – Stimulating the SP channel can facilitate the transportation and transmutation of body essence, and build up qi and blood.
- **Kidney channel** (KI) – pertains to the kidney system. As base of the life, it balances the body's yin and yang.
- **Urinary bladder channel** (UB) – tai yang channel; connects the entire internal organ system. Stimulating this channel can regulate zang fu system.
- **Large intestine channel** (LI) – contains more qi. Activating this channel can help detoxify the body, clearing heat toxins.

Most of the points used for facial rejuvenation acupressure routines are on one of the above six channels. Some are "extra," or Ashi, points.

The following are the main facial rejuvenation acupressure points located on the face: Yang Bai (GB14), Tong Zi Liao (GB1), Feng Chi (GB20), Si Zhu Kong (SJ23), Cheng Qi (ST1), Si Bai (ST2), Ju Liao (ST3), Di Cang (ST4), Ying Xiang (LI20), Xia Guan (ST7), Jia Che

(ST6), Quan Liao (SI18), Jing Ming (UB1), Zan Zhu (UB2), Shang Xing (DU23), Bai Hui (DU20), Tai Yang (extra point), Yin Tang (extra point), Qiu Hou (extra point), Yu Yao (extra point).

Here are other commonly used body points for facial rejuvenation acupressure: Zu San Li (ST36), Feng Long (ST40), San Ying Jiao (SP6), Yin Ling Quan (SP9), Xue Hai (SP10), Guang Ming (GB37), Qu Chi (LI11), Yang Xi (LI5), He Gu (LI4), Tai Chong (LIV3), Chi Ze (LU5), Yang Liao (SI6), Fei Shu (UB13), Xin Shu (UB15), Ge Shu (UB17), Gan Shu (UB18), San Jiao Shu (UB22), Da Zhui (DU14), Ming Men (DU4), Tai Xi (KI3).

Acupressure Manipulating Techniques

With acupressure, the hand or fingertips are the tools used to activate points along the channels. There are many different hand techniques for performing acupressure. The simplest one, the only one we will use in this book, is a special type of pressing and kneading. This is a one-finger acupressure technique, usually using the pads of the index finger and/or thumb to press on the chosen point or knead it in a to-and-fro motion. You can simply call it digital pressing motion. This motion should start lightly and gradually increase; the overall effect should be soft, yet penetrating.

The rate of pressing, for this book's purpose, should be 60–100 times per minute. You can press rather quickly, at a rate up to 100 pressings per minute, or slower, depending on the conditions you are treating.

Cautions and Contraindications for Acupressure

Do not use patient acupressure on your patient if he or she has any cardiovascular, brain, or lung condition; contagious skin condition; bleeding problems; or is feeling full or hungry. If your patient is pregnant, apply acupressure with caution by avoiding working on the following points: GB21, LI4, SP6, SP10, UB60, UB67, LIV3, and any point on the lower abdomen, upper abdomen, or lower back.

Chapter 12
Facial Acupressure Protocols

As discussed in previous chapters, all yin and yang channels meet in the face. Because the face is where the energy merges, the treatment of the face is very important.

The acupressure facial protocols introduced here are based on the channel theory and include three types of manipulation:

1. Massage used according to the drainage pathway of the lymphatic system, which helps to detoxify the body
2. Point pressure used on the acupuncture points to regulate the function of meridians, open qi and blood flow, and create lusterous skin and a rosy complexion
3. Massage used according to the muscle pattern to recover muscle tone, tighten the skin, and prevent wrinkles

The skill of the practitioner is very important in facial acupressure. He or she should practice qi gong breathing while focusing attention on accurate acupressure manipulation. Consistent, even, and soft pressure that penetrates the superficial layer of the skin should be applied during the whole procedure for the best results.

The following is a comprehensive facial acupressure protocol. This protocol promotes qi and blood flow to the face, lifts sagging of the face, smoothes wrinkles, helps lessen facial discolorations and age/dark spots, and treats eye concerns such as dark eye circles, puffy eyes, and eye bags. Most importantly, it calms and anchors spirit. I divide the facial area into several regions according to the different concerns or purposes of the protocol.

1. Nasal Area (See Fig. 12.1 on page.248)
Helps clear sinus that causes dark circles and eye bags; clears heat from the face; smoothes wrinkles
- Start on the Yin Tang point using direct digital pressure. This helps calm the patient at the start of the treatment.
- Then stroke bilaterally from UB2 down to LI20, and stroke back up to UB2. This helps to open up the nasal passage. Repeat this 3–5 times.

2. Side of Face (See Fig.12.2–12.5 on pg.248-249)
Clears away stagnation; lifts sagging of chin; promotes lymph drainage; smoothes wrinkles
- Begin at Yin Tang using the thumbs, and stroke bilaterally to Tai Yang.
- Use direct digital pressure on Tai Yang 3 times.
- Then, with the pads of the thumb, move from Tai Yang to SJ21, SI 19, and GB2, using direct digital

pressure on each point 2–3 times (See Fig.12.2 on page. 248).

- Massage the ear and gently pull down on the earlobe. Massage up to the ear apex and gently pull up on the ear apex (See Fig. 12.3 on page.248).
- Start again at Yin Tang and, with the pads of the thumbs, gently stroke over the eyebrows to Tai Yang and down in front of the ear to ST5. Press the ST5 3–5 times.
- Then stroke down to ST9 and very gently press ST9 2–3 times (See Fig. 12.4 on page.249).
- Begin again at Yin Tang and stroke to Tai Yang, then up to GB8 and down the hairline to GB20. With the thumb on GB20, place the index finger on Tai Yang and press 2–3 times.(See Fig.12.5 on page.249).
- Pull up the neck and gently center the patient's head.

3. Eye Area (See Fig.12.6–12.10 on page.249-251) 、
Treats dark circles and eye bags; smoothes wrinkles around eyes (claw's feed); lifts up sagging of eyes; brightens eyes.

- Have the patient close his or her eyes and, using the thumb pads, gently press on the eyes, from inside to outside. Then gently press on the lower and upper eyelid, repeating 3–5 times on each stroke. (See Fig.12.6 on page.249).
- Place the index, middle, and ring fingers, respectively, on UB2, Yu Yao, and SJ23. Apply

gentle digital pressure 9–12 times (See Fig. 12.7 on page.250).

- Place these same three fingers, respectively, on the ashi point of the lower eyelid (below the inner canthus of eye), ST2, and another Ashi point (below the outer canthus of eye). Apply gentle digital pressure 9–12 times (See Fig. 12.8 on page. 250).
- Using the thumb and index finger, gently squeeze above the eyebrow (just over UB2, Yu Yao, and GB1) and on upper eye lid (UB1, ST1, and Qu Hou on lower eye lid). Repeat 3–5 times (See Fig. 12.9 on page.250).
- Finish the eye area protocol by using both middle fingers gently massage upper and lower eyelid with the patient's eye closed (See Fig.12.10 on pg.251).

4. Trigger Points on the Face

Promotes deep blood flow and lymph drainage; helps collage production process.

Using the thumb and index finger at the same time, press the following pairs of points:

- ST8 with ST3
- GB14 with SI19
- ST6 with ST7
- SJ17 with ST4
- ST6 with LI20

5. Lifting Sagging of the Face, Chin, and Neck (See Fig. 12.11–12.12 on page.251)

- Stroke from Yu Yao to GB14, then down the stomach channel through to ST7 and ST6, then up to ST4, ST3, ST2, and back to Yu Yao. Repeat 3–5 times (See Fig. 12.11 on page.251).
- For neck wrinkles: Stroke from ST9 to SJ17. Repeat 3–5 times (See Fig. 12.12 on page.251).

6. Upper Facial Area and Top of Head (See Fig. 12.13–12.15 on page.252)

Lifts the face; firms and smooths wrinkles

- Press on DU20 and extra points Si Shen Cong. Repeat 3–5 times.
- Using the pads of the thumbs, stroke from Yin Tang to DU23, from UB2 up to UB5, from Yu Yao to GB14, and then up to UB4. Next, stroke from Tai Yang to ST8. Repeat 9–12 times (See Fig. 12.13 on page.252).
- Using the thumb pads, sweep from center of the forehead outward to Tai Yang area. Repeat 9–12 times (See Fig.12.14 on page.252).
- Using light flicking with the index finger, tap from front hairline to top of the head along DU channel, then from front hairline along UB channel, finishing from Tai Yang up along GB channel. Repeat 3–5 times (See Fig.12.15 on page.252).
- Using the index and middle finger, press on GB20 9–12 times, then gently grasp GB21 6–9 times.

- Finish with rubbing the palms together 36 times and, without touching the face, massage over the entire face with the palms of the hands (qi gong style).

Section 5
Traditional Chinese Dietary Therapy for Facial Rejuvenation

Chapter 13
Introduction to Chinese Dietary Therapy
for Facial Rejuvenation

As early as 2,000 years ago, and probably much earlier, Chinese texts lauded the beautifying effects of many foods. The famous TCM physician, Bian Que, during the Warring States period, stated, "If a person is diseased, he should be treated with food first. If food treatment fails to work, then use herbs." The herbal bible, *The Divine Husbandman's Classic of the Materia Medica* (*Shen Nong Ben Cao Jing*), which dates from the Han dynasty, documented more than 50 different foods, many of which have effects that enhance facial beauty. Foods such as Chinese dates, long yan rou fruit, red beans, grapes, apricot seed, etc., have already been mentioned. Just as Chinese herbs in concentrated form promote healing, certain foods, when emphasized therapeutically, benefit the Three Treasures in addition to providing nutrition. Food therapy, as much as other TCM techniques in facial rejuvenation, is a powerful tool for smoothing wrinkles, diminishing dark eye circles, eye bags, and facial discoloration, among other conditions.

Food Types, Chinese Style

Like Chinese herbs, each food has its own properties. Each has a distinguishing flavor, a temperature, a channel it enters, and a therapeutic function.

The flavor of the food (sweet, pungent, sour, bitter, or salty) has very important application to its healing effects. Sweet foods, for example, tonify qi and blood, nourish yin, and moisten dryness. Sweet foods refresh the skin and have an anti-aging effect that improves dry, wrinkly skin. Pungent food has a dispersing effect, which is good for superficial skin conditions. Bitter food detoxifies the skin. Sour or astringent food improves oily skin. Salty food expels skin nodules.

Temperature is another important food property for facial beauty. Cold food, for example, clears heat from the skin, cools the blood, and detoxifies. Thus, it can be very helpful for treating heat-induced skin conditions like acne, rashes, and spotting. Remember, though, that "cold" food isn't literally cold as though it just came out of the freezer. "Cold" is a descriptive term for a property of the food's "nature."

Color is another way of categorizing food for targeted facial beauty benefits. There are five colors for food:

- **Red:** According to TCM's five-element theory, red goes with the heart. Red foods help improve the skin's complexion. They usually enter the heart channel, and have an anti-aging effect. Beneficial red foods include tomatos, red rice, carrots, strawberries, and watermelons.

- **White:** White foods enter the lung channel—white being the color of the lungs. They nourish the skin, and are best if you have fair skin prone to dryness. Beneficial white foods include tremella, coconuts, bamboo, pears, water chestnuts, and lotus root.

- **Green:** Green foods are associated with the liver, which governs the free flow of emotions. Green foods relax the body. They also moisten and cleanse the skin. They are often anti-inflammatory, that is, anti-infection. Recommended green foods include cilantro, field mint, bitter melon, kiwis, dandelions, green apples, fresh luffa, asparagus, and all kinds of bitter greens.

- **Black:** Black foods belong to the kidneys. They delay the aging process and rejuvenate the skin by tonifying the kidney system and the blood. Beneficial black foods include black beans, black sesame seeds, black fungus (Chinese name: Hei Mu Er), black mushrooms, black Chinese dates, blackberries, mulberry fruit, seaweed, and other sea plants

- **Yellow:** Yellow foods enter the spleen channel and nourish the entire body and its energy. That includes the skin and face. Beneficial yellow foods include yellow soybeans, millet, ginger, papayas, bananas, and pineapples.

One of the food goals will be to include foods in daily meal plan of different colors and flavors. That will ensure beneficial foods entering different channels and boosting different organ systems. Some foods work best for certain facial conditions, in the appropriate chapters.

What Foods Do for You

Foods have specific healing actions. Choosing an adequate variety of foods in the diet promotes the following actions and effects. Depending on one's condition, however, one or more foods should be emphasized.

- Expel wind: This action helps treat itchy skin, red rashes, acne, and facial discoloration.
- Tonify the body: It is important to tonify yin and yang, qi and blood. This action is beneficial for treating wrinkles, dry skin, withered and dull complexion, dark eye circles, puffy eyes, eye bags, and sagging.
- Drain the dampness: This action is good for a puffy face, eye bags, dark eye circles, as well as skin discoloration, dull complexion, and acne.
- Transform phlegm: This action helps eye bags, eye puffiness, a red swelling nose (especially the tip of the nose), rough skin, dull complexion, and facial dark spots.
- Expel stasis: This action helps dark spots, age spots, rough skin, a dull and dark complexion, and dark eye circles.
- Regulate qi: By regulating energy, certain foods can improve dark spots, aging spots, dark eye circles and eye bags.

Food Suggestions for Different Skin Types

Oily skin:
Mung beans, different berries, bitter melon, lemons, grapefruit, apples, grapes, celery. These astringent (sour) foods help decrease sebaceous secretions.

Dry skin:
Tremella, honey, pears, olives, cabbage, honeydew melon, bananas. These foods provide water to help moisturize and nourish the skin.

Normal skin:
Watermelon, cucumber, onion, mushroom. These foods maintain the pH balance of the skin and promote metabolism.

Anti-aging foods:
Red vegetables and fruits, red peppers, tomatoes, carrots, watermelon, red peaches. All of these are directed to the heart channel, which promotes regeneration of skin cells and prevents aging of the skin, thus brightening the skin.

Chapter 14
Anti-wrinkle/Anti-sagging Foods
in Traditional Chinese Medicine

Chances are most people have never even heard of some of the foods on the following list, let alone tasted them. But they have all been found by TCM practitioners to have a profound effect on the prevention of wrinkles and sagging. These foods should be part of a regular diet to keep the face as smooth as possible.

1. Bird's Nest
This Chinese delicacy and health food is exactly what it sounds like—the edible abode of birds called swiftlets that fashion their nests using the male's saliva. Available as a food or supplement in Chinese grocery stores or by mail order, bird's nest is considered one of the most precious nutritional aides for beauty and rejuvenation.

Its specific wrinkle-smoothing properties come from its action on the skin and lungs, its ability to moisturize, and its support of the body's immune system. Modern research has found that bird's nest contains epidermal growth factor (EGF), which is a water-soluble glycoprotein, as well as vitamins and minerals.

2. Chinese Dates (Jujube Fruit)

This fruit's medicinal value has been recognized in China for 4,000 years. There's even an old Chinese saying that "three dates a day keeps old age away." The special function of these dates is to generate energy and blood to nourish the skin, promoting a healthy glow and smoothing wrinkles. Rich in antioxidant vitamins and minerals, it is the ideal fruit (fresh or dried) to moisten dry skin and lips. Make sure to take the pits out of the dates before you eat them.

3. Black Sesame Seeds

These little black seeds are anti-aging wonders that, in TCM terms, nourish the internal organs, the blood, and body fluids in general. As such, long-term, regular consumption of black sesame seeds is especially effective fighting wrinkles resulting from dry skin conditions. From a Western point of view, the seeds are rich in plant protein, vitamin E, and linolenic acid, all essential for healthy, wrinkle-free skin.

4. Peanuts

There's a reason peanuts are a staple in Chinese cooking. TCM literature refers to peanuts as "ever-live fruits"—meaning they have an anti-aging effect when eaten regularly. Peanuts fight wrinkles by nourishing the lungs and strengthening the stomach and spleen. Western nutritionists have recognized the value of peanuts, which are rich in readily absorbable amino acids, with a protein concentration (about 30%) nearly equal to chicken, eggs, and red meat. Though they contain fat, peanuts actually help lower cholesterol levels. One caution: Make sure any peanuts you eat are fresh, because old or spoiled peanuts may contain carcinogenic toxins. Choose high-quality, organically grown peanuts.

5. Black Soybeans

There is a traditional Chinese text called the *Yian Nian Mi Lu* that focuses on anti-aging secrets. The text raves about how soybeans benefit facial complexion. According to TCM, black soybeans promote tissue growth, replenish bone marrow, tonify deficient organs, and moisturize the body. As is well known in the West, soy is one of the best sources of plant protein. It is rich in natural estrogens known as isoflavones; essential fatty acids, including omega-3; vitamin E; and several important minerals. For best results, choose black soybeans, or soy products made from the black soybeans.

6. Pig Skin

It may not be the Western idea of a healthy food, but the Chinese discovered long ago that pig skin is an "herb" that nourishes yin, relieves irritability, and is used effectively for dry and wrinkled skin based on the ancient Chinese medical theory that "like heals like."

According to modern science, pig skin (fresh or dried) contains basic nutrients that our skin needs in order to delay wrinkle formation. It has abundant protein, mainly gelatinous protein and fibrous protein (collagen fiber, elastic fiber). It's also rich in minerals and the vitamins B1 and B2. The fat content of the pig skin is only half that of pork meat itself. Moreover, pig skin has a cell structure similar to human skin, with a very compatible kind of protein (large-cell protein). All of these qualities make pig skin an important food for delaying the skin cell aging process, for softening and beautifying skin, and for reducing and preventing wrinkles. It is usually available from any local butcher.

7. Walnuts

Walnuts are another time-honored Chinese "treasure" for nourishing the complexion and smoothing facial wrinkles. They are among the ingredients of many ancient Chinese herbal formulas for beauty. Walnuts are recognized in the West as being very nutritional. They are rich in cholesterol-lowering unsaturated fats and omega-3 fatty acids, linolenic and oleic acids, the antioxidant carotene, vitamins B1 and B2, and a number of other natural anti-aging substances.

A handful of walnuts every day will do well. However, one might want to start with walnuts using this ancient Chinese protocol: Eat 1 piece each before going to bed for 5 nights. Then start eating 2 for the next 5 nights. Every 5 days, add another walnut until you reach 20.

8. Cherries

Cherries are energizing foods that beautify the skin by nourishing the spleen and stomach (the middle jiao).

Because of their high iron content, they are a wonderful skin-smoothing fruit that improves skin color as they enrich the blood. They are so effective that, besides eating them, one can simply crush cherries and apply the juice directly to your face.

9. Honey

If your daily sweet treat is honey, then you will find over time that your will power is heightened, your body is "enlightened," your aging process has slowed down, and your face is less wrinkled. Honey tonifies energy and calms the five internal organs. It's a superb skin nourisher, and its unique antibacterial and antiviral capabilities help protect skin cells.

Honey is rich in vitamins, amino acids, organic acids, complex carbohydrates, hormones, proteins, fructose, and glucose. The skin easily absorbs many of these nutrients, making honey an excellent food for nourishing the skin as well as improving skin function and regeneration.

TCM considers honey to be an herb as well as a food, and its anti-wrinkle benefits can be enjoyed in supplement form and included as part of meals. One way is to simply swallow a teaspoon of honey each morning on an empty stomach, like (very sweet) medicine. Or mix a teaspoon of honey and a teaspoon of vinegar in 6 ounces of water and drink half of that mixture at a time. Be sure to use only pure, organic honey.

Honey can also be used as a great facial mask. Combine 1/4 teaspoon of honey, 3 drops of olive oil, and

1/2 teaspoon of pearl powder. Mix it well in the palm of your hand with some water and apply it to your face once every other day. Wash it off with warm water after 20 minutes. Amazing results can be seen from first-time use.

If sugar intake is a concern, try substituting royal jelly for honey. It's not sweet and it's less sticky. This is an especially beneficial food for women with low sex drive and wrinkled skin. Use it as you would use honey but with a low dosage of 1/4 teaspoon daily.

Caution: Some people are allergic to bee products. If you know or suspect that you have such an allergy, don't use honey, royal jelly, or any other bee product. If an allergic reaction occurs (such as rashes or wheezing) upon using a bee product, discontinue use immediately and see a physician.

10. Tremella

Tremella is a mushroom that has long been used in China for general skin beauty, both as a food and as a supplement. But it's a do-all food that nourishes lung yin, increases energy, and benefits the blood, brain, heart, and immune system. And its yin-nourishing function makes it especially beneficial for those with dry, wrinkled skin who also suffer bouts of irritability or who are going through menopause. It is rich in vitamin D and minerals, including iron, sulfur, phosphate, magnesium, calcium, and potassium.

Tremella is made in an already prepared form, with sugar added, which is available at health food stores or Chinese markets. However, it is better to buy the actual mushrooms (they will be cultivated, not wild) at a Chinese market.

One convenient way to prepare tremella is as follows: Soak 2 ounces of tremella mushrooms overnight. Then section them by hand into small pieces, throwing away the yellowish part at the bottom. Simmer slowly in 75 ounces (about 9 cups) of water for 2 hours 30 minutes. Or use a pressure cooker, adding 5 measuring cups of water, keeping a mid-boil going for about 30 minutes. When it's cooked, add 2 teaspoons of honey and let cool. Keep the cooked tremella in a glass jar in the refrigerator, eating about 1/2 cup worth each morning.

More Great Anti-wrinkle Foods

There are considerably more than ten ways to utilize dietary therapy to combat wrinkles. Get in the habit of including the following foods in a regular diet. They all have natural healing properties that include wrinkle prevention and facial smoothing. Most of these foods are readily available; a few may need to be purchased in Chinese markets.

Pine nuts
Sea cucumber (sometimes called "Ginseng from the sea" because of its high nutritional value)
Lotus root
Pork or chicken cartilage (boil it as a soup)
Pork bone (boil it as a soup)
Fish (all kinds)

Squid (or calamari)

Lingon berries

Wild yam (also an herbal supplement)

Chinese cabbage

Luffa (the fresh form of the same plant that serves as a scrubber or massager)

Tomato (it's also a detoxifier)

Cucumber

Seabuckthorn

Black mushrooms

Reishi mushrooms

Olive oil

Coix seed

Bee pollen

Euryale

Foods That Detoxify

The strong belief in Traditional Chinese Medicine that our body is able to detoxify itself when given the chance is directly relevant to the wrinkle-smoothing quest. The accumulation of toxins in the body upsets internal balance, contributing to wrinkling. The following foods energize the body's natural detoxification systems, helping to rid the bloodstream and organs of toxins and beautifying the skin. They should become part of one's regular diet.

Green Tea

Green tea is well known in Chinese medicine as a super detoxifier, and in Western medicine as a super antioxidant—two ways of saying the same thing. Green tea is loaded with antioxidants in the form of polyphenols, flavonols, vitamin E, vitamin C (four times more than in lemons), carotene, and much more. That antioxidant effect (100 times more than vitamin C alone) protects the skin from the damage caused by the sun's ultraviolet rays, toxic food additives, secondhand tobacco smoke, and stress. A good way to take advantage of green tea's detox power is to combine it as an infusion of one of the anti-wrinkle herbs given earlier. Remember, though, that it contains caffeine, so limit intake and try to drink it only in the morning if one tends to get "hyper" with caffeine. Do not drink green tea against the advice of your doctor.

Bitter Melon
Fresh bitter melon can be found in Chinese or other Asian markets (as a juice or a supplement in liquid extract form). It is nutrient-rich and is thought to stabilize blood sugar levels. More important, bitter melon contains properties that, in TCM terms, clears away heat, relieves lethargy, sharpens the eyes, and nourishes the skin. If buying the whole fruit, wash it and remove the seeds, then boil it in soup or cook as a dish.

Niu Bong
Also known as burdock root, this vegetable is used to detoxify the body, especially the blood. It contains trace minerals, foliate, vitamins C and B, and amino acids. Buy it fresh in Asian markets. Wash one long stick and cut off some to add to soup or boil to make a tea.

Coix Seeds

Coix seeds resemble large barley. They benefit the skin by strengthening the digestive system, leeching out dampness, and detoxifying the body. They can be found at most herb stores or Chinese markets. Mix them with rice or in a soup.

Pomegranate

This fruit benefits and detoxifies the digestive system.

Black Fungus

Used throughout the centuries as a body cleanser and detoxifier, this wonderful food/herb has such powerful cleansing properties of the digestive system that Chinese workers often use it to offset occupational contamination hazards. It is rich in vitamins, minerals (especially iron), and proteins. It will help clear wrinkles. Buy it at an herb store or Chinese market. Soak it in hot water until it spreads and softens, boil, and include in soups, salads, or just about any main dish. We also discuss black fungus in chapters dealing with weight loss and age spots.

Lotus Root

It's a delicious food/herb and available at Chinese markets. Wash the root, dice it or cut it into small pieces, and use it raw in salads or include it in soups. The lotus root will clear heat, moisten the lungs, cool the blood, benefit the digestive system, enlighten the body, beautify the skin, and delay the aging process.

Celery

Clears heat; promotes urination.

Garlic

Kills parasites.

Seaweed

Cleanses the body; softens nodules.

Chapter 15
Foods for Facial Discoloration and Dark/Age Spots

A major part of TCM facial rejuvenation regimen includes a diet consisting of certain foods that have been shown for thousands of years to help brighten and even out facial complexion. Beyond their nutritional value, the foods recommended in this chapter provide a therapeutic effect on the body's internal blood and qi flow that will be reflected on the face.

Food therapy for facial rejuvenation adheres to the basic tenet of Chinese medical philosophy, which holds that external beauty is a mirror reflecting internal health. These foods help address the internal imbalances that result in a spotted or discolored complexion. Of course, their beneficial effect is gradual, and, for best results, the food therapy program must go hand in hand with the other complexion treatments—herbs, acupressure, and qi gong.

Some of the best foods that the Chinese associate with a good complexion are so common that you will be surprised at the benefits they hold. Some other foods are more exotic and might require a little poking around in Chinese or Asian markets. There is no strict regimen to follow with these or any other skin-saving foods. You should recommend the use of these foods to your patients in their regular meal planning.

Dong Gua (Winter Melon)

This gourd vegetable and its seeds are known as a healing herb, but it's also a very popular health food in China, especially as a soup. It benefits the heart, detoxifies the body, and beautifies the skin. Whether eaten as a food or taken in herb form, dong gua improves complexion by removing wind from the skin.

Winter melon is an especially worthwhile addition to one's diet if one is having complexion problems, eye bags, or dark eye circles. Eating it regularly also helps to lose weight.

Finding winter melon throughout most of the year in Asian markets or even in Western-style organic food stores should be no trouble. It's also called wax gourd or white gourd. Eat it as any melon, peeling off the outer skin. Remove the seeds and pulp, but save them for topical use for an even more radiant and spotless skin.

Shi Gua (Luffa)

You may only know this vine plant from the sponges made from the fibers inside the overripe fruit, but the young vegetable is a traditional food in China and one of my favorites for keeping my complexion young looking. It enters and clears the liver and stomach channels, and contains such skin-nourishing phytochemicals as lycopene and carotene.

These zucchini-like vegetables can easily be grown if space is available. They are also available at Chinese markets. Prepare them as any squash. It also makes an excellent topical mask for dealing with wrinkles, dark spots, and uneven facial discoloration.

Bai Luo Be (White Turnip)

This is a fairly common turnip, often called daikon, which offers plenty of medicinal benefits. In TCM terms, bai luo be is acrid, sweet, and cool in nature, entering the spleen and lung channels to detoxify the body and free up stagnating fluids in the channels. I've observed a definite beneficial effect on the complexion when bai luo be is eaten regularly. The best way to use it for facial discoloration is to juice it every morning and drink about a half cup.

Shi Zi (Persimmon)

Most people know about this delicious fruit, but rarely eat them. To reduce dark spots on face, they should be eaten often. Shi zi has been known for centuries to clear heat from the body, nourish the lungs, and moisten the skin—all actions that improve one's complexion. They are also rich in vitamins C and A, potassium, calcium, and iron. The leaves of the plant are also used as herbs.

You may find two different kinds of persimmons. The Chinese version of the fruit is sometimes known as kaki. Both the Chinese and the American persimmons are great for the complexion. They can be eaten, but make sure they are very ripe. Don't eat the skin. Dried persimmons are a special treat that might be found in Chinese markets. Another way to use persimmon to brighten the complexion is simply to apply the fresh peel to the face.

Sang Shen Zi (Mulberry Fruit)

The recommendation of herbal extracts of mulberry as a wrinkle-reducing treatment has already been presented. Now try eating the mulberry fruit itself, called sang shen zi, to help clear and brighten the complexion. Mulberry trees have a long history in Chinese medicine. They are used to raise silkworms, which eat the leaves as their main source of nutrition. Dried silkworm is an excellent complexion herb.

The fruit of the mulberry isn't a true berry, but it is berrylike in taste and appearance, and contains beneficial antioxidants also found in blueberries, raspberries, and the like. One plant chemical (phytonutrient) found in mulberry fruit and berries, called cyanin, is responsible for the red or purplish color and is thought to have a strong therapeutic effect. From a TCM point of view, sang shen zi is a blood tonic that benefits the yin and kidneys, helps overcome weakness, and brightens a withered-looking complexion as well as clearing dark spots from the face.

Mulberry fruit is sweet tasting and a little tart, and can be eaten as any berry. If raw fruit itself cannot be found, try searching the Web or local health food stores for fresh raw mulberry juice.

Bai Guo (Ginkgo Nut)

The health benefits of ginkgo leaf extract have been widely discovered in the West. Much modern research indicates that the antioxidant plant chemicals in ginkgo benefit blood flow, and may even slow memory loss.

Not many are aware that in Chinese medicine, the nut of the ginkgo tree is more often used medicinally. While ginkgo nut extract is used by herbalists, the whole nut itself, often roasted, is a traditional Chinese food that nourishes lung energy and calms wheezing. Its health benefits show up in one's complexion, which will become noticeably cleaner and clearer if ginkgo nuts are a regular part of your diet and facial applications. To use ginkgo to clear the complexion topically, simply crush the fresh nuts into a paste and apply directly.

Yi Yi Ren (Coix Seed)

You've already met this wonderful seed, which derives from a barleylike grain, as a beneficial food for smoothing wrinkles and clearing the eye area. But it deserves special mention here for its ability to clear up discoloration of the facial complexion, especially age spots and other dark spotting.

Coix seed is a better protein source than most other grain seeds, and it is rich in vitamins. It is a very effective strengthener of the digestive system. Coix oil is very good for the skin. It's easy to find in Chinese markets. It can be eaten almost daily simply by sprinkling 12–15 grams of the raw seed in soup.

Eggs

Chicken eggs are considered a superior herb/food in Traditional Chinese Medicine, with a surprising variety of beneficial effects. As a food, eggs anchor the heart and calm the five organ systems. The whites clear heat from the lungs, detoxify the body, and nourish the skin. Those actions help brighten the face, smooth wrinkles, and clear away dark spots. The yolks tonify the blood, helping to rejuvenate a withered, pale complexion, which is often the result of blood deficiency.

Eggs should be eaten once per day for a person with a healthy, balanced lifestyle. If a lot of saturated fats are not included in diet, the body can then handle the cholesterol in eggs without harm. If there one does have a cholesterol problem, eat just the whites. A good way to eat eggs is to put beaten eggs in soups, especially soups with luffa and tomatoes.

Another common use of eggs is as a topical beauty product. If there appears to be discoloration on the face and dry skin, apply raw, beaten yolk and white together. If one has oily skin, use just the egg white as a mask.

Feng Mi (Honey)

The ancient Chinese Daoists lauded honey as a superior herb that calms the five organs and nourishes qi. They believed honey was capable of relieving hundreds of diseases, with the ability to harmonize the actions of hundreds of other herbs ingested into the body.

A little bit of honey every day is recommended. A teaspoon in warm water or with one's favorite tea will work just fine. Regular, long-term honey use strengthens will power and "enlightens" the body to prolong life. It also promotes a radiant, rosy complexion, making the face, according to one text, "as beautiful as a flower."

If you want to try something even more potent than honey, try royal jelly instead. Use it orally or topically. Use only 1/4 teaspoon in warm water if you're going to drink it down. Topically, apply royal jelly every night and wash it off the next morning.

Remember, though, that if allergic to bee products, one should not use honey or royal jelly internally or topically. To know for sure, take just a tiny bit internally, or apply a dab to a small area on the inner side of your wrist. If there is any reaction, don't use it again.

Shan Yao (Chinese Yam)

Chinese yam is considered a main course in China, not a side dish. It's eaten as much for its medicinal properties as its taste. Shan yao is sweet, warm, and neutral. It tonifies heart energy; strengthens the stomach, spleen, and lung systems; and nourishes kidney qi. All those actions benefit the skin and hair, promoting a radiant facial complexion and helping to eliminate discoloration and dark spots.

Fresh Chinese yam is easy to find, and should be eaten often. For variety, buy dried yam at a Chinese market and include 6 to 9 grams in your soup. You can also grind the dried yam into a powder and add it to whatever flour you bake with.

Other Foods That Are Great for Facial Discolorations and Dark/Age Spots

Tomato: Use as a soup stock, or juice it and drink. It's also very effective as a facial application.

Eggplant: Simply cut it into small pieces and rub it on the dark spot until the area is slightly reddened. Leave the area unwashed for an hour. Do this every day for 10 days.

Mung Bean: Cook it as a bean soup or grind it into a powder to make a facial mask for dark spots and discoloration.

Black Bean: Eat it often prepared in soup, or cook it first and add it to salads or other dishes.

Peas: Big green peas can be cooked any style you like. Also mash them into paste and apply topically.

Cucumber: It's great cooked, raw, in soups, or applied topically.

Chinese Cabbage: Cook it any style, or juice it to include in a vegetable juice cocktail. It's also good applied topically.

Water Chestnuts: Juice or cook with other ingredients.

Chapter 16
Food Therapy for Eye Rejuvenation

Food therapy does for the eyes exactly what herbs do, that is, they balance the internal organ systems to achieve an inner health that is reflected in clear youthful eyes.

Foods for Eliminating Dark Eye Circles

If dark eye circles are the main problem, look for the following foods at a good health food store or a Chinese market. They directly address stagnation and kidney yin deficiency that are often the inner cause of those unsightly discolorations.

Try to include as many of these foods as possible in the meal plan, and as often as possible. Later in this chapter you find some ideas for using many of these foods in delicious recipes that are based on Chinese tradition.

Hei Mu Er (Black Fungus)

This is a common food among the Chinese people, a staple in just about every vegetarian dish. One should have no trouble finding Hei Mu Er at any Asian market, good health-food store, or herb market. Make sure you buy true Chinese black fungus and not just any dark mushroom.

Used throughout the centuries as a detoxifier, this wonderful food/herb has such powerful cleansing properties that Chinese workers often use it to offset occupational contamination hazards. In TCM, it's considered a "sweet," neutral herb (though it doesn't taste sweet) that enters the stomach and large intestine channels to tonify body energy and promote blood flow. Because it is rich in vitamins, minerals (especially iron), and proteins, and is such an effective cleanser of the digestive system, it is also one of the best foods to clear the area around the eyes of dark circles and wrinkles.

Hei Mu Er is simple to prepare. Simply soak the fungus pieces in hot water until they spread and soften. Rinse clean and boil. Include them sliced in soup or salads, or add them to any hot dish.

Chi Xiao Dou (Azuki Bean)

Here is one of the best and easiest steps to take to help get rid of dark eye circles. Simply substitute this reddish, oval bean for whatever kind of bean you usually prepare as a side dish. Chi Xiao Dou is an ancient Chinese bean that's been popular in the Orient for thousands of years, and it's readily available in North America.

As common as this bean is, few foods are better for rejuvenating the eye area. Chi Xiao Dou has ideal properties for healthier eyes. It enters through the heart and small intestine channels to clear dampness out of the body as it eliminates toxicities, strengthens the digestive system, moves blood stagnation, and relieves swelling. That all makes it an effective food for eliminating dark eye circles (and puffy eye bags, as well).

Prepare Chi Xiao Dou as you would any dry bean. Soak overnight in clean water, drain, rinse, and simmer until soft, using about 4 cups of water for every cup of beans. If one forgets to soak them overnight, unsoaked beans will cook in about 15–20 minutes in a pressure cooker.

Dao Zao (Chinese Dates)

One of the all-purpose herbs used in Traditional Chinese Medicine, Dao Zao is wonderfully effective for clearing up discoloration in the eye area. Chinese date porridge is strongly recommended to anybody having trouble with dark eye circles.

Dao Zao rejuvenates the eye area by strengthening the digestive system, which in turn generates abundant qi via the postnatal sea of energy. It also improves blood flow. The overall effect of eating Chinese dates regularly is increased nourishment in the eye area and a reduction in swelling around the eyes. Remember to take out the pits inside the dates.

Foods for Helping Eliminate Eye Bags and Puffiness

Here are three foods to include in the diet if puffy eye bags are making the eyes look tired and old. Each food addresses the organ imbalances most often related to eye puffiness. Specifically, each helps correct the dampness accumulation caused by spleen qi deficiency. And each helps remove the "fatty ball" type of eye bag—what Western medicine might call a fat deposit but what TCM considers to be phlegm obstruction.

Kun Bu (Kelp Thallus)

A big difference between Oriental and Western diets is the liberal use of sea vegetables that the Chinese, Japanese, and other Asians eat. The most valuable sea vegetable for reducing eye puffiness is a kind of kelp called kun bu. If eaten regularly, it will clear out phlegm congestion and reduce dampness accumulation and the swelling that goes with it.

Kun bu can be found in food markets that carry Asian specialities. (If not available, any other dark "seaweed" will be an acceptable substitute.) Buy it dried, usually in thin strips, soak it in hot water for several hours and then simmer it to make a broth. Or boil it for just 10 minutes and use the cooled and chopped kelp as a condiment or garnish. Dry or fresh, kun bu is something that can be eaten almost daily. Sprinkle it on salads or add some to any main dish without altering the main flavor too radically.

Carp Fish

From the TCM point of view, fish varies not just in taste and texture but in the healing properties they impart. For eye rejuvenation, carp is king of the sea. As it clears away heat and detoxifies the body, carp addresses the causes of eye puffiness by strengthening the digestive system and reducing swelling from dampness accumulation. For the eyes' sake, try to eat carp at least once a week, preferably more often.

Yi Yi Ren (Coix Seed)

Reader was introduced briefly to these barley seeds in a number of wrinkle-reducing recipes. This all-purpose skin beautifier is even more valuable as an eye-rejuvenator. The main reason for yi yi ren's effectiveness is that it helps clear dampness from the body, thus reducing swelling. But coix seeds are also excellent for the digestive system. And they're easy to add to just about any dish.

Healthy Foods to Brighten and Energize the Eyes

Even without eye bags or dark circles, eyes may tend to look tired and spiritless. Vision may blur on occasion, or eyes tear up. These symptoms, especially if they tend to occur after straining oneself physically or emotionally, usually mean that the liver blood is deficient and kidney essence is depleted. Because the liver channel opens to the eyes and kidney essence nourishes and replenishes the eyes, weakness in those organs spells trouble for the eyes.

Fortunately, there are plenty of foods that help improve the situation. Following are some of the most powerful. Work some of them into the meal plan each day and noticeable progress toward regaining healthy eyes will be seen. Many of them are also recommended for dark circles and puffiness.

Yams
Carrots
Fish
Walnuts
Chrysanthemum flower
Liver (beef)
Mulberry fruit
Millet
Almonds
Soybeans
Seaweed
Lotus root
Apricots
Sesame seeds
Sunflower seeds

Section 6
Other Effective Modalities
for TCM Facial Rejuvenation

Chapter 17
Qi Gong Exercises for Facial Rejuvenation

Qi Gong: Mind, Body, and Breathing

Qi gong may be less familiar than herbs or acupressure, but it's actually considered the highest level of self-healing for facial beauty. It is actually an older practice than herbal medicine, a unique treasure of Traditional Chinese Medicine.

The purpose of qi gong is to assist the body's natural self-balancing capacity by manipulating internal energy with one's mind and breathing. Like acupressure, it involves no introduction of outside elements (such as herbs or food). But it is even more self-sufficient than acupressure because you don't even need to press anything. All the "work" is done with the mind, the breath, and some gentle movement.

Qi gong uses the body by moving it. It uses the breath by concentrating it and directing it in specific ways. And it uses the mind by focusing it to achieve relaxation and to move energy.

Using qi gong to promote beauty and slow down aging is not a new variation. It has been a beauty treatment for thousands of years. Of course, it is a whole body exercise that helps essence, qi and spirit. It incorporates TCM concepts of yin/yang, the five elements, channel theory and the organ systems.

Qi gong has been influenced by Chan, or Zen, ("sitting") meditation, which was heavily influenced by Daoism. It regulates the heart (which rules the emotions), purifies the spirit, and promotes the free flow of qi.

Principles for Successful Qi Gong

Qi Gong is not physically difficult. But it is probably unlike anything your patients have tried before. Much of it involves using the imagination to move energy around in the body.

If you decide to introduce qi gong exercise to your patients as part of their daily facial rejuvenation exercise, inform them it can take some practice to feel comfortable doing that. Let them know that, if they stick with it, before long it will become easy.

Here are some suggestions for doing the exercises. Refer back to these when the actual exercise instructions appear.

The body position: There many different body positions involved in qi gong. But almost all the exercises given will simply require sitting comfortably in a chair. A hard chair is best. Keep body upright, relax the shoulders, let both hands rest loosely on the lap, set feet at shoulder-width on the floor, and let them just relax.

Breath: Breath, above all, should be even. Even breathing is best achieved by keeping it natural yet softer than normal breath. Sometimes one might find themselves short of breath or even "forgetting to breathe" because focus is on something else. If that happens, stop everything and relax. Figure out what caused the problem and start over. After some practice, soft, even breathing will come naturally.

Mind: Qi gong exercises are mind exercises. You will be using your mind to concentrate on your body or a part of it. You will also be using your mind to create energy. Imagining energy balls or energy movement is a big part of qi gong. The secret, as you might have guessed, is relaxation. Focusing first on soft, even breathing helps you relax; so does repeating a relaxation word of your choice, such as "calm" or "relax." Sometimes one will be asked to focus the mind on an actual channel point, as in acupressure. Usually these are points on the middle or lower parts of the body. One such such point is called the dan tian. It is located 2 cuns (or 2 thumb widths) directly below the navel.

The following is a qi gong exercise used a lot both by me and by my patients at home. For more qi gong exercises for facial rejuvenation, refer to my book *Anti-Aging Therapy: How to Clear Away Your Wrinkles and Rejuvenate Your Face.*

The Energy Ball

This is a wonderful 15-minute, four-step qi gong exercise that energizes the face to rid itself of wrinkles, sagging of the face, dark/age spots, facial discoloration, dark eye circles and eye bags. It is based on using the power of imagination to create healing energy in the form of an "energy ball." Though it starts in the mind, the energy ball is quite real and full of body essence and qi that will help beautify the face and take care of its wrinkles.

In this exercise, focus your attention on an area about 2 inches below the naval called dan tian, which will be your energy ball's home. The energy ball will be "sent" on a route that will take it along the REN channel (conception channel) that runs right up the center of the torso to the upper lip. It will also follow the DU channel (governing channel) that runs from below the coccyx area up to the spine, passing the vertex of the head, descending along the middle line of the face and stopping at the inner upper lip.

Start by sitting in a chair, eyes lightly closed and mood relaxed. Focus on your breathing, keeping it slow, even, and natural for about a minute. Then follow these four steps:

Step 1: Concentrate on the dan tian area for half a minute, holding both hands on the dan tian area, palms facing it. Then begin to imagine a small energy ball, about the size of a Ping-Pong ball, coming together there. Visualize its form

and energy. Use your imagination to "exercis
making it become smaller and bigger in the d

Step 2: Now imagine sending this energy ball via the REN channel (conception channel) up the front middle line of the trunk to the top of your head, then down the governing channel along the middle line of your back. Return the ball back to the dan tian. Let this energy ball circle around the REN and DU channels for 5 cycles before having it come to rest again in the dan tian.

Step 3: The energy ball has now acquired healing power. Use the power of imagination to breath in the essence of the clear sky and fertile land (that is, from heaven and earth), imagining these vital nature essences entering through the opened skin pores, nourishing and replenishing the skin. Bring the breath all the way down to the dan tian. Then imagine the pores opening wide as you breathe out the accumulated toxicity from the face. Repeat this breathing technique 5 to 10 times until feeling a slight heat sensation or dampness in your face. Concentrate your attention in your dan tian area as you finish.

Step 4: Use the hands to draw out the energy ball from the dan tian, imagining it exiting in the form of a stream of light.

Step 5: Now move the energy ball with both hands up to your face, separating the ball into two half-balls, one in each hand.

Step 6: Massage the forehead area with these half-balls of energy, one on each hand, with palms (about 1 inch away from the face) facing the area of the forehead that needs to be worked on. Use 10 circular motions.

Step 7: Using the same motion, massage each side of the face simultaneously (one half-ball on either side). Imagine the wrinkles being ironed flat while completing 10 circular motions. Do this without actually touching the face; keep hands about an inch away.

Step 8: Massage the wrinkled areas around the eyes with the energy half-balls, giving each side 10 slow circular massage motions. Imagine your eyes brightening, wrinkles smoothing out, eye bags disappearing, dark circles fading, face firming, sagging lifting up. Focus on the area where your wrinkle concerns are.

Step 9: Bring the energy half-balls back down to the dan tian area, uniting them into a full energy ball again. Exercise the energy ball with palms facing together; make it smaller and smaller in front of the dan tian area.

Step 10: Slowly reinsert the energy ball into the dan tian, again in the form of a stream of light. Take three deep breaths to finish the session.

Chapter 18
Cupping for Facial Rejuvenation

Cupping is a technique commonly used in TCM practice for stimulating local blood flow and clearing stagnation by using the suction from small cups placed on the body.

In ancient China, cupping was as a widely used form of folk medicine. Cupping was originally called jiao fu, which means "animal horn," because in ancient times, people used animal horns as cupping instruments.

As early as the Han dynasty, the famous Daoist Ge Hong, in his famous medical book *Emergency Formulas in the Sleeve* (*Zhou Hou Bei Ji Fang*), documented cupping treatment for furuncles (boils) using a cow's horn. After much development and refinement, today cupping is commonly used in TCM practice in conjunction with acupuncture and acupressure (tui na) protocols.

According to TCM, cupping treatment can achieve the following functions:
- Move qi and invigorate the blood
- Warm channel and unblock the stagnation
- Reduce swelling and alleviate pain
- Expel dampness and relieve cold

- Drain the heat and expel toxicity

In TCM facial rejuvenation, cupping can be used to move qi and blood, and release the toxicity from the body. Specifically, it is beneficial for conditions of dark/age spots, facial swelling, sagging of the face, rough skin, and dull complexion.

There are different kinds of cups used at different times for different purposes. The most commonly used cupping instrument is glass cups. There are also plastic cups that do not need to be heated.

There are different sizes of cups. For TCM facial rejuvenation purposes, medium- to small-size cups are ideal.

1. For dark/age spots and facial discoloration
Procedure: cupping LI11, SP10, UB17, UB22

2. For dark eye circles and eye bags
Procedure: cupping Tai Yang, UB17, UB18, SP10

3. For wrinkles
Procedure: cupping UB13, UB15, UB18, UB21

4. To release the body's toxicity
Procedure: cupping UB 13, UB 17, UB 40
Procedure (alternate): Move the cup along UB channel from UB 10 to UB 25. Repeat 3 times. (Make sure put ointment on the skin surface when using this moving cupping technique.)

Precautions and Contraindications for Cupping

Cupping is contraindicated for the following conditions: bleeding problem, skin infection, ulcer, contagious skin conditions, eczema, high fever, convulsions. Do not use cupping on the abdomen or lower back area of a pregnant woman, on the large blood vessels, or on the chest near the heart.

Chapter 19
Gua Sha for Facial Rejuvenation

Gua sha technique refers of the use of the fingers or a small board with smooth edges to massage, manipulate, and stimulate certain points along the channels of a particular area in order to promote qi and blood flow, and remove toxins from the body. There are different kinds of gua sha hand techniques for different body conditions. This book emphasizes the gua sha method called "scrape," which involves applying a gentle, soft, and steady force from a gua sha board over the skin surface. Depending on body conditions, there are often bruise marks left on body surface from gua sha treatment. They normally disappear in several days. Under normal circumstances, there are not any bruises left on the face after treatment, because much gentler force is applied. However, patients given gua sha treatment should be informed before the treatment of the possible side effects, including bruise marks, even on the face.

Gua sha is different from other TCM modalities in that it uses oil or cream to enhance treatment effectiveness and to lubricate the skin to reduce pain caused by the procedure. There are different kinds of gua sha oils and creams for the different conditions. For the purpose of this book, a natural, nutritional skin healing cream is needed for gua sha facial rejuvenation procedures.

Gua sha treatment is an effective, commonly used modality in TCM facial rejuvenation that not only promotes qi and blood flow but also helps the skin better absorb nutrients from facial or eye cream.

Gua sha is commonly used for TCM facial rejuvenation concerns such as wrinkles, sagging, dull complexion, discoloration, dark/age spots, dark circles, and puffy eyes. Below we introduce basic gua sha procedures that are used for different facial concerns:

1. Wrinkles and sagging of the face

Gua sha on the face

Step 1: Apply an anti-wrinkle cream to the face, massaging it into the skin for 1 minute. Open up the wrinkle with one hand, and hold the gua sha board in the other. Using the round point of gua sha board, apply cross-wrinkle friction (meaning the motion of the gua sha stroke is perpendicular to the wrinkle lines) several times on each set of wrinkles, especially on any channels points that happen to pass the wrinkles. Work on the whole wrinkle line with gentle yet steady force. The wrinkle area should look slightly red from gua sha. Figure 19.1 (See page.254-255) shows specific techniques for different wrinkles on the face.

Step 2: After working on each set of wrinkle lines, use the flat edge of the gua sha board to "iron the wrinkled area flat."

The facial area can be divided into three regions according to where the wrinkles are located. Each region has its own gua sha procedure.

Forehead region: Starting gua sha from the middle of the forehead, one finger fix the center of forehead where your gua sha board starts, the other hand holding gua sha board, gently scrape from middle toward outside. Repeat 6–12 times, then change to the other side of the forehead (See Fig 19.2 on page. 255).

You can also use both hands performing gua sha together. With both hands holding a gua sha board, start from the middle line of the forehead. Working towards out and stop until the gua sha boards hit side of hairline. Repeat 9–12 times.

To lift the face, place left hand on the forehead toward the front hairline, as if pulling the forehand upward. Then with the right hand holding the gua sha board, scrape straight from ying tang to DU23, then from Yu Yao through GB14 to GB 15. Finish by scraping from SJ23 to ST8. Repeat 6–12 times (See Fig 19.3 on page. 256).

Cheek region: This area covers the cheek area between the eyes and mouth. Imagine drawing lines from the center of the face (nose area) out and upward towards the side of the face. Gua sha direction should follow these imagined lines.

If you perform one hand gua sha, you can start from one side by using one hand lifting and hold the skin at the side hair line, then use another hand holding the gua sha board and gently scrape the skin along the imaging lines from nose area out and upward towards the holding hand at the side of the face (See Fig 19.4 on page. 256). Or you can also place the holding hand near the nose over the skin while the other hand holding gua sha board performing gentle gua sha strokes from middle of the face near the nose towards side of hairline (See Fig 19.5 on page 256). Repeat 9–12 times and followed by gua sha on the other side of the face with the same procedure and hand techniques. If you choose to use both hand, perform gua sha at the same time, then simply hold both gua sha board in each hand starting together from the middle (on either side of the nose), using even, gentle and steady force up and outward. Repeat 9–12 times.

Chin region: This covers chin area and front neck area. Imagine drawing lines from the center of chin and front center of the neck going up and outward towards jaw area and SJ17 area (for the neck). Using same gua sha techniques as used in second region (See Fig.19.6 on page. 257). Repeat 9–12 times.

Caution: Gua sha on the face should always be gentle. It should create a light red reaction on the skin, but not leave bruises like those from gua sha on the body.

Gua sha on body

There are two channels used for body gua sha:

1. GB channel—Starting from GB 20, scrape along GB channel to GB 21. Make sure the strokes go in a one-way direction. Repeat 9–12 times.

2. UB channel—Starting from UB 10 to UB 17, one-way direction, repeat 9–12 times.

2. Dark eye circles, eye bags, and puffy eyes

Gua sha on the face

Step 1: Apply eye cream to the eye area. Gently perform gua sha along the lower eyelid, from inner side of eye, near Bi Tong, towards the Tai Yang area. Use very gentle strokes in a one-way direction (See Fig. 19.7 on page. 257). Repeat 3–5 times. Then start the very gentle gua sha stroke along the upper eyelid from UB1 to Yu Yao, to Tai Yang. Repeat 3–5 times.

Step 2: For claw's feet: With one hand, gently spread out the wrinkled area and the other hand holding the gua sha board. The procedure should be done in two steps: First, scraping outward along where the claw's feet are and gently "iron the wrinkles flat" (See Fig. 19.8 on page. 257). Repeat the procedure 5–7 times. Do one side at one time. Then keeping spreading the wrinkles open with one hand, and with gua sha board on the other hand, scraping outward with a spiral motion over the wrinkled area (See Fig 19.9 on page. 258). Repeat 6 times. Caution: the strokes must be very gentle so as not to cause bruises.

Gua sha on the body

Back: Gua sha from UB17 to UB23, one side at one time, in one direction. Repeat 9–12 times.

Front: REN 12 to REN4 in one direction. Repeat 9–12 times.

Leg: Starting from SP6, move upward to SP10. Repeat 6–9 times. Then perform local gua sha on SP6 and SP10 against the channel flow. Repeat 9 times.

To perform gua sha on a local point, simply scrape through the point in a one-way direction. The direction depends on the condition being treated. If a point needs to be supplemented, then the stroke goes with the channel flow. If the point needs to be drained, then the stroke goes against the channel flow. Either way, it does not affect gua sha's effectiveness in promoting the flow of qi and blood, and detoxification.

3. Facial discolorations and dark/age spots

Gua sha on the face

Step 1: Using the wider side of the gua sha board, scrape from the jaw area up to the ST2 area. Make sure the gua sha board covers the entire cheek area (See Fig.19.10 on page.258). Do one side at a time, or both sides together. Repeat 9–12 times.

Step 2: Locate where the dark/age spots are. Then, starting from the local spot area, scrape outward in different directions. Repeat 6–9 times (See Fig 19.11 on page.258).

Gua sha on the body

Back: Gua sha from UB11 to UB23, one side at one time, in one direction. Repeat 9–12 times.

Leg: Start from SP6 and go upward to SP10. Repeat 6–9 times. Then perform gua sha locally on SP6 and SP10. Repeat 9 times.

Arm: Start from LI11 and go downward to LI5. Repeat 6–9 times. Then perform gua sha locally on LI11 and SJ5. Repeat 9 times.

Cautions and contraindications for gua sha:

- Before beginning gua sha treatment, caution the patient about the possibility of bruising and inform him or her of the contraindications.
- Because the gua sha may produce bruises, the force of gua sha should be gentle, but even and steady. Extra caution should taken when performing gua sha on facial area, which is most prone to bruising.
- Gua sha is contraindicated for the following conditions: hemophilia or any other blood disease, skin irritation, any growth on skin, bone injury, contagious skin condition, very weak body constitution, chronic disease, blood vessel ailments, pregnancy.

Chapter 20
Moxa for Facial Rejuvenation

Moxa is a very common treatment used with acupuncture treatment to enhance its effectiveness. There are different moxa treatment methods, such as direct moxa, indirect moxa, pole moxa (moxa stick), warm-needle moxa (moxa put on top of needles), etc. In TCM facial acupuncture, moxa stick and indirect moxa are often used.

Basically, moxa is used to warm and unblock the channels, move qi and promote blood flow, warm the middle and tonify qi, and strengthen the body system. Moxa treatment enhances acupuncture treatment in facial rejuvenation for specific cold and deficiency conditions:

For wrinkles
Condition: qi and blood deficiency
Procedure: moxa REN12, REN6, ST36

Condition: kidney deficiency
Procedure: moxa REN4, KI3, SP6

For sagging of the face
Condition: spleen qi deficiency
Procedure: moxa DU20, REN6, ST36

For eye bags or dark eye circles due to deficiency conditions
Conditions: Spleen qi deficiency with phlgm obstruction; kidney yin deficiency; qi and blood stagnationic
Procedure: moxa REN6, REN12, UB17, UB18, SP10

Cautions and contraindications for moxa
Moxa is contraindicated for heat and excess conditions. Do not use moxa on the abdomen or low back of pregnant women. Do not use moxa on the head or face of patients with high blood pressure, headache, or fever.

Section 7
Comprehensive TCM Treatments
for Facial Rejuvenation

Chapter 21
Root and Branch Treatments
for Special Facial Concerns

Note: In the following sections of this chapter, many Nefeli herbal supplements and topical skin care formulas are mentioned as treatment suggestions. Please refer to Chapter 10 for details.

21.1 Wrinkles

Identifying Different Types of Wrinkles

One type of wrinkles is caused by temporary skin dehydration. This type of wrinkle usually is shallow and thin, distributed around the eye, mandible, and/or corner of the mouth. Skin tone is lusterless due to lack of fluids. These wrinkles can occur at any age due to dry skin. They are easily treated.

Another type of wrinkles is caused by qi and blood deficiency. These shallow wrinkles tend to be distributed around the eyes, lips, and forehead. They may occur on after an illness or giving birth. They are moderately easy to treat.

Another type of wrinkles is due to aging and essence deficiency. These deep wrinkles (extending to dermal area) tend to be distributed as eye crow's feet, around the mouth, forehead, cheek, and neck area. Treatment can be prolonged, due to the slow recovery rate.

There are different stages of wrinkle formation:

- Stage 1: Skin dryness. Wrinkles might not yet be visible.
- Stage 2: Lusterless skin; loss of elasticity. Minimum wrinkles are seen.
- Stage 3: Loss of skin tone. Shallow wrinkles begin to appear.
- Stage 4: Deep wrinkles form.

TCM Pattern Identification and Root Treatment

1. Heart Blood Deficiency

When the heart blood fails to nourish the skin, thin shallow wrinkles will occur with a lusterless complexion, pale tongue, thin pulse, and blurred vision.

TCM Root Treatment:

- Acupuncture: UB15, UB17, UB20, ST36, SP10
- Herbal Treatment: Si Wu Tang (Four Things decoction), Ba Zhen Tang (Eight Treasures); or Nefeli Complete Balance and Nefeli Wrinkle Smoother.
- Food Therapy Suggestions: lamb, walnuts, mushrooms, soybeans, Chinese dates, cherries, carrots, beets, red grapes, bee pollen, honey

- Topical Application: Nefeli Intensive Wrinkle Care Day Cream, Nefeli Intensive Wrinkle Care Night Cream, Nefeli Facial Rejuvenating Mask

2. Qi Stagnation and Blood Stasis

Suppressed emotions cause liver qi stagnation, which impedes free flow of qi and blood in the channels. As a result, wrinkles occur due to the blockage of qi and blood. Other signs and symptoms include fatigue, irritability, and irregular menstrual cycle.

TCM Root Treatment:
- Acupuncture: LIV3, LI4, UB18, UB17, ST36
- Herbal Treatment: Xiao Yao San (Rambling Powder) combined with Nefeli Complete Balance and Nefeli Wrinkle Smoother
- Food Therapy Suggestions: lotus seed, citrus peel, chrysanthemum, flower, peach flower
- Topical Application: Nefeli Intensive Wrinkle Care Day Cream, Nefeli Intensive Wrinkle Care Night Cream, Nefeli Facial Rejuvenating Mask

3. Kidney Essence Deficiency

Kidney essence deficiency is the major cause for the aging process. It is reflected by the skin (as part of the body system) with signs of sagging and wrinkles.

TCM Root Treatment:
- Acupuncture: REN4, KI 3, SP3, SP6, LIV3, UB18, UB23

- Herbal Treatment: 6 Rehmannia, Nefeli Complete Balance, Nefeli Wrinkle Smoother
- Food Therapy Suggestions: yam, lotus root, ox tail, ginseng, Gou Qi Zi, Wu Wei Zhi
- Topical Application: Nefeli Intensive Wrinkle Care Day Cream, Nefeli Intensive Wrinkle Night Care Cream, Nefeli Facial Rejuvenating Mask.

4. Spleen Qi Deficiency

When spleen qi is deficient, its function of transportation and transformation will be significantly impeded. As a result, the face will be malnourished, resulting in sagging facial skin, puffy eyes, and at times dark brownish spots on the face.

TCM Root Treatment:

- Acupuncture: REN4, ST36, REN12, SP3, SP6
- Herbal Treatment: Eight Treasures, Ren Shen Yang Zoung Wan (Ginseng Decoction to Nourish the Nutritive Qi), Nefeli Complete Balance, Nefeli Wrinkle Smoother
- Food Therapy Suggestions: ginseng (substitute American Ginseng for patients with high blood pressure), Bai Mu Er (tremella), walnuts, peanuts, tomatoes, lotus root, Dang Sheng, yams, cinnamon powder
- Topical Application: Nefeli Intensive Wrinkle Care Day Cream, Nefeli Intensive Wrinkle Care Night Cream, Nefeli Facial Rejuvenating Mask

5. Irregular Lifestyle

Smoking, alcohol consumption, sleep deprivation, and greasy high-fat food can all add toxins to our body, which will affect healthy qi and blood flow. As a result, our face will suffer from dark discoloration, wrinkles, and other unhealthy conditions. Educate patients to regulate their lifestyles. They should eat healthy foods and try to keep a balanced emotional state.

Branch Treatment for Wrinkles

Depending where the facial wrinkles are distributed, local treatment can be given accordingly:

- Remember, when needling on the wrinkles, it is called Ashi treatment.
- The common way to enter the needle is to first, go along with wrinkles, and needle the beginning and ending point of the wrinkles.
- Second, choose the nearest points on a particular channel that happens to be passing through or near the wrinkles. The directions of the needles need to be upward to achieve a lifting effect.

1. Wrinkles on the Forehead

Points to use:

- Needle ST8. Pull up the skin and hold with one hand, then insert the needle with the other hand. Angle the needle upward at 45°.

- Needle GB15. Pull up the skin and hold with one hand, then insert the needle with the other.
- Needle Yin Tang. Use the the same lifting technique as described above.

Distal points: GB34, GB41, GB43

2. Wrinkles Above the Eyebrows
This area primarily involves the stomach and gallbladder channels.

Point to use: GB14, to activate blood in the channel
Distal points: GB34, GB41, ST44

3. Wrinkles Along the Tai Yang Area (Temples)
This area primarily involves the gallbladder and stomach channels.

Points to use: ST 8, Tai Yang
Distal points: GB 34, ST 44.

4. Crow's Feet
Points to use: Tai Yang, GB1, SJ23. – Use the lifting technique with ½-inch needles, insert on a 45° angle; or use intradermals.

Distal points: Use according to the specific diagnosis.

5. Wrinkles Between the Medial Ends of the Eyebrows
Where the DU and urinary bladder channels pass,

Points to use: UB2; Yin Tang and DU3, with needle upwards.
Distal points: UB40, UB60.

6. Neck Wrinkles

Points to use: GB20, SJ17, ST10, ST9.

7. Lip Wrinkles

Points to use:

- Open and pull the skin outward while needling DU26 and REN23.
- Needle ST4, using a 45° angle upward.

8. Wrinkles Around the Nose

This is governing, stomach, large intestine channel involvement.

Points to use: SI19; ST4; ST7; LI20; Yin Tang with needle upward; if the nose is red, add with DU25 to clear heat in the nose.

Distal points: LI4, the command point of the face; ST3; ST44; LU7

9. Wrinkles in Cheek (Zygomatic) Area

This area involves the stomach and small intestine channels.

Points to use: ST2, SI18

Distal points: SI6; Yang Lao; HT3, which brings rosiness to the cheeks coupled with ST9.

10. Wrinkles Anterior to Ear

This involves the stomach and San Jiao channels.

Points to use: GB2, SJ22, ST7, ST9

Distal points: ST36, SJ5, SJ6, or SJ7—all of which send energy to the face

11. Wrinkles Around the Mouth

This involves the stomach channel.

Points to use: ST5, ST6, ST7

Distal points: LU7, ST36, LI4, ST44, GB 34, GB 41, DU 26, REN 23

12. Wrinkles Around the Mandible/Jaw Bone

This involves the stomach channel.

Points to use: ST5, ST6, ST7

Distal points: LI4, ST36, ST44.

CASE STUDY

A 56-year-old woman complains of increased wrinkle formation on her forehead and sagging facial skin, especially on her cheek area. Other complains include insomnia, dry skin overall, and a tendency to be easily stressed. Her pulse was thin and weak in kidney positions; tongue was slightly pale, with a comparatively red tip.

Diagnosis:

Kidney essence and liver blood deficiency. When kidney essence is deficient (as her pulse suggested), the body tends to age more. This can be manifested as sagging face and increased wrinkles, a formation due to the decrease of cell turn over in the skin. Insomnia and pale tongue signify the patient has liver blood deficiency. When the blood is deficient, it fails to nourish the face, and fails to anchor the spirit. As a result of this, the winkle condition will be worse.

Treatment Principles:

Replenish liver and kidney essence; firm and lift the face; smooth the wrinkles.

Treatment:

- Acupuncture Root Treatment: KI3, UB15, SP6, ST36, LI10
- Acupuncture Branch Treatment: DU20, SI18, Ashi points (points where the deepest wrinkles are located)
- Explanation: UB5 and SP6 are used here to nourish the liver and heart blood so it can anchor the spirit and at the same time readily make sure of the blood flow to the facial area to replenish the cells in the face. KI3 nourishes kidney essence. ST36 is used to build up qi and blood, so when the blood is nourished qi has to be able to push the blood flow. LI10 (or LI9 depending on which is more sensitive for the patient) is used for wrinkle conditions. On the face, DU20 lifts the upright qi for sagging of the face. SI18 works as a motor point for firming the skin and activating blood flow in the face. Reinforced needle technique on body points is applied here. Moxa is done for 2 minutes each on UB23 and ST36.
- Herbal Suggestions: Nefeli's Wrinkle Smoother herbal supplement is prescribed for the patient. Major herbs in this formula include Ginseng, Dang Gui, E Jiao, Guo Qi Zi, Tu Si Zi, Ling Zhi. Dang Gui is included for nourishment of the blood and to promote blood flow, particularly to the facial area. E Jiao aids liver blood. Ling Zhi calms the spirit. Gou Qi Zi and Tu Si Zi

together provide an age-reversing facial boost, typically for wrinkle conditions. Ginseng tonifies qi and lifts sagging of the face.

- Food Therapy Suggestions: organic lamb and Gang Gui stew twice a week; 3 Chinese dates each day; 2 oz pig skin (obtain from local butcher; scrape away all the fat; cut it; and cook in soups) every day.
- Topical Skin Care Suggestions: Nefeli Intensive Wrinkle Care Day Cream, Nefeli Intensive Wrinkle Care Night Cream, Nefeli Facial Rejuvenating Mask

After the first acupuncture treatment and the use of Nefeli Facial Rejuvenation Mask, the patient noticed immediate results on her face: The wrinkles in her forehead and smile lines were much shallower. Her face looked firmer and lifted. The skin showed a healthy glow instantly.

By the second week, the patient's face showed healthier glow. The forehead wrinkles were significantly smoothed. The patient experienced an increase in energy, and her sleep was getting progressively better.

After 10 sessions (sessions were given twice per week), the facial wrinkles were much smoother. The jaw line became more permanent, suggesting firmness of the facial muscles. The patient was told to continue using Nefeli Wrinkle Smoother and Nefeli Complete Balance to continue nourishing liver and heart blood, tonifing kidney essence, and balancing the body's yin and yang. The patient was also given Nefeli eye cream and mask to combine with anti-wrinkle treatment.

Facials were given during the treatment period. The patient started an exercise routine and lost more than 10 pounds. With the anti-wrinkle treatment protocol she was on, the sagging and wrinkles on her face continued to decrease, making her look much younger.

21.2   Double Chin/Sagging Face

TCM Pattern Identification and Root Treatment

1. Spleen Qi Deficiency

The spleen has a special function for holding muscle and flushing in place. This function is done by abundant spleen qi, which is supported by the body's essence. When the spleen's transportation and transformation function is low, it fails to generate the needed body nutrients, resulting in low energy (qi deficiency). As a result, the face will be malnourished, which manifests as sagging and puffy eyes.

TCM Root Treatment:

- Acupuncture: REN6, REN12, DU20, ST36, SP6
- Herbal Treatment: Bu Zhung Yi Qi Tan decoction, which tonifies the middle and benefits the qi; Nefeli Complete Balance; Nefeli Wrinkle Smoother
- Food Therapy Suggestions: ginseng, huang qi, lotus seed, yam,
- Topical Application: Nefeli Facial Rejuvenating Mask, Nefeli Intensive Wrinkle Care Day Cream, Nefeli Intensive Wrinkle Care Night Cream

Branch Treatment:

This involves the San Jiao and stomach channels.

Points to use: ST6, ST10, ST11, SJ17, REN22, Jia Lian Quang (extra point 1 cun lateral to REN22), SJ7, ST44, SP9; electronic stimulation on ST6 and Jia Lian Quang.

CASE STUDY

A 60-year-old woman complained of sagging face and double chin, which she had had for more than 10 years. Recently, however, it had been getting worse. The patient complained of weak legs and knees, and low energy at times. The pulse showed kidney and spleen deficiency. The tongue was pink with light white coating.

The patient's condition was due to aging, where the organ system, especially kidney system, becomes deficient. It manifests in weak legs and knees. Low energy is another result of deficient organ functions, especially the spleen and stomach systems.

TCM Diagnosis:

Kidney essence and spleen qi deficiency causing collapse of muscles and skin.

TCM Treatment Principle:

Tonify kidney essence; tonify and raise spleen qi; lift sagging of the face.

TMC Treatment:

- Acupuncture Root Treatment: DU20, REN4, REN6, ST36, GB34, UB40, UB20 (optional)
- Acupuncture Branch Treatment: ST8, UB6, DU23, REN23.

ST36, GB34, and UB40 are the three leg yang lower He-Sea points. Activating these lower He-Sea points can increase the yang qi on the face to give lift. REN6 is where the source of body's essential resides. It strongly tonifies and promotes flow of qi. DU20 lifts the face (Caution: skip this point if patient has a history of high blood pressure or suffers from excessive headaches. Use a supplemental method.) ST8, UB6, DU23, and REN23 are points on specific channels that run through the face. Activating these points helps promote free flow of qi and blood in local channels on the face. For lifting purposes, the following hand manipulation should be followed:

- ST8: Make sure the needle points upward.
- UB6: Using index finger, press on UB1 and glide the finger all the way up along the UB channel with a steady force to UB6. Enter needle on UB6 pointing upward.
- DU23: Using index finger, press on DU25 (tip of the nose) and glide the finger all the way up along DU channel to DU23. Enter the needle upward.
- REN23: Enter needle upward. Before the acupuncture treatment, 10 minutes of facial acupressure is given to lift the face to move qi and blood circulation in the face. After the acupuncture session, Nefeli Facial

Rejuvenating Mask is applied on the face, followed by Nefeli Anti-Wrinkle Night Cream.

- Herbal Treatment: Nefeli Wrinkle Smoother—to tonify kidney essence, tonify and raise spleen yang qi, and nourish liver blood to support the qi movement
- Food Therapy Suggestions: fish, especially catfish; red beans; yam; lotus seed; Ginseng
- Topical Application: Nefeli Facial Rejuvenating Mask, Nefeli Intensive Wrinkle Care Day Cream, Nefeli Intensive Wrinkle Care Night Cream

Patient was instructed to perform facial massage protocols once a day, with Nefeli Intensive Wrinkle Care Day Cream as the massage cream.

Patient received facial acupuncture 8 times over a one month period, along with herbal supplements and facial acupressure. Her face and chin area were significantly lifted by the end of treatment.

21.3 Eye Bags and Dark Circles

TCM Pattern Identification and Root Treatment

1. Blood Stagnation

Blood stagnation is the major cause of dark eye circles.

TCM Root Treatment:

- Acupuncture Treatment: UB17, UB18, UB20, SP6, SP10. For eye bags, add SP9, ST40, and moxa ST36. For dark eye circles, add SP10, LI11.
- Herbal Treatment: Nefeli Eye Refresh herbal supplement
- Food Therapy Suggestions: animal liver, eggs, carrots, apricots, sunflower seeds, sesame seeds, black fungus, Chinese dates
- Topical Application: Nefeli Essential Eye Care Cream, Nefeli Eye Rejuvenating Mask

2. Phlegm Obstructing Channels

This is the main cause of eye bags.

TCM Root Treatment:

- Acupuncture Treatment: UB20, ST40, SP9, SP6, LI4
- Herbal Treatments: Si Jun Zj Tang (Four Gentleman decoction), Nefeli Eye Refresh
- Food Therapy Suggestions: seaweed, citrus peel, radish, chives, carrots, apricots, sunflower, sesame seeds, black fungus, Chinese dates, turnip, tomatoes, orange, lean meat, pumpkin
- Topical Application: Nefeli Essential Eye Care Cream, Nefeli Eye Rejuvenating Mask

3. Liver and Kidney Yin Deficiency

Long-term liver and kidney yin deficiency creates stagnate heat. When this heat becomes chronic, it will congeal in the channel system, especially in the area under the eyes where the skin is very delicate and thin. As a result, dark circles will occur.

TCM Root Treatment:

- Acupuncture Treatment: KI3, LIV3, UB18, UB23, SP6
- Herbal Treatment: Liu Wei Di Huang Wan (Six Rehmannia decoctions), Nefeli Eye Refresh
- Food Therapy Suggestions: pears, sea cucumber, bird's nest, tremella, carrots, apricots, sunflower, sesame seeds, black fungus, Chinese dates, turnip
- Topical Application: Nefeli Essential Eye Care Cream, Nefeli Eye Rejuvenating Mask

TCM Branch Treatment:

DU23, Yu Yao, GB14, GB1, Tai Yang, ST2. For eye bags, add ST2 or ST3. For dark eye circles, add ST7.

CASE STUDY 1

A 58-year-old male complains of low energy, an obstructed feeling during urination, eye puffiness, and eye bags. His pulse was weak and slippery in the Guan and Chi positions in both hands. The tongue body was dark, with a light gray to white coating.

TCM Diagnosis:

Dampness obstruction in the middle and lower jiao, with underlining kidney essence and spleen qi deficiency.

This was the condition, with dampness obstruction in middle and lower jiao was manifested by the obstructed urination and slippery pulse. Underlining kidney essence and spleen qi deficiency was manifested by fatigue and weak pulse.

TCM Treatment Principle:

Transform dampness from middle and lower jiao, replenish kidney essence, strengthen spleen, and reduce swelling.

TMC Treatment:

- Acupuncture Root Treatment: REN12, REN6, REN3, ST28, SP6, ST36, LIV3
- Acupuncture Branch Treatment: UB2, Yu Yao, GB14, ST3.

REN12, REN6, REN3 are major points in the conception vessel that strongly tonify the body's yuan qi (especially REN 6), transform phlegm from middle jiao (REN12), and clear away dampness obstruction from lower jiao (REN3). ST36 supports qi and blood, especially up to the facial area as the lower he-sea point of the yang ming channel. LIV3, as a yuan source point of the liver channel, nourishes liver blood and promotes blood flow at the same time.

During the treatment, serine needle manipulations were performed: supplement on ST36 with needle pointing upward (9 times); strong stimulation on SP6 with needle turned upward until patient felt sensation increase (9 times); clockwise stimulation on REN12 and REN6; counter-clockwise stimulation on REN3.

The patient received immediate results after 25 minutes of treatment. He had urination without any obstructed feeling. The eye bags were totally diminished under right eye and 50 percent diminished under left eye.

- Herbal Treatment: Nefeli Complete Balance and Nefeli Eye Refresh were recommended to harmonize his liver and kidney, tonify spleen qi, and drain dampness.
- Food Therapy Suggestions: yam, beats, turnip, carrots, black beans, carp fish, seaweeds

CASE STUDY 2

A 45-year-old female complains of puffy eyes and severe dark circles under her eyes. She tended to become very stressed. Her period was infrequent but with several PMS symptoms: mood swings and bloating in her chest and abdominal area. Sometimes she felt feverish right before the period. Her eating habits were irregular, and she had a feeling of being tired all the time. She also suffered from sinus conditions. According to the patient, the dark eye circles got worse with emotional stress and sinus conditions. Her pulse was thin, wiry, and slippery. Her tongue was dark with a white coating.

TCM Diagnosis: Liver qi stagnation with spleen qi deficiency. The constrained liver qi made the patient suffer from PMS and stagnation of blood flow, which can be a cause of dark eye circles. Stress, an irregular lifestyle, plus liver qi stagnation affect the spleen function. All of these give rise to eye puffiness and dark eye circles. Her on-and-off sinus conditions were due to spleen deficiency. Stress contributed to her dark eye circles.

TCM Treatment Principle: Soothe the liver; promote qi and blood flow; strengthen spleen function; promote local qi and blood flow in the eye area.

Treatment:
- Acupuncture Treatment: LIV3, LI4, ST36, SP6, SP10
- Acupuncture Branch Treatment: Tai Yang

The four gates at the yang source point of the large intestine and liver channels promote free flow of qi and blood, and soothe liver qi. SP6 is used here as a hormone balancing point. SP10 promotes blood flow, moving blood stagnation from eye area. ST36 tonifies qi and blood, and promotes qi flow to facial area.

- Herbal Treatment: Xiao Yao Wen, Nefeli Complete Balance, Nefeli Eye Refresh, Nefeli Cold and Allergy Care to help treat and prevent her sinus conditions
- Food Therapy Suggestions: Fu shou fruit (Chinese vegetable for soothing constrained liver qi), Chinese dates, black fungus, dark green leafy vegetables
- Topical Application: Nefeli Essential Eye Care Cream (patient reported that when first applying cream, she experienced a slight tingling sensation, which then faded. The cream is designed to work that way.); Nefeli Eye Rejuvenating Mask (to enhance the treatment).

After three treatments and using all the modalities recommended for two weeks, patient's dark eye circles dramatically lessened, and eye puffiness totally disappeared. She felt much calmer. Her sinus condition cleared up.

21.4. Facial Discoloration and Dark/Age Spots

TCM Pattern Identification and Root Treatment

This condition is closely related to liver, spleen, and kidney organ functions.

1. Liver Qi Stagnation
Facial discoloration and dark/age spots are yellowish and brownish in color, and often worse before menstruation. When liver qi is stagnated, it will cause blood to stagnate leaving dark spots and discoloration on the skin.

TCM Root Treatment:
- Acupuncture: UB18, UB17, LI11, LIV3, LI4, SP6, SP10
- Herbal Treatment: Nefeli Bright Complexion, Shao Yao Wan
- Food Therapy Suggestions: Chinese cabbage, Fu Shou fruit, fried whole wheat, chrysanthemum, fresh luffa fruit, tomatoes, winter melon, strawberry, kiwi, green pepper, eggs, dark greens

- Topical Application: Nefeli Facial Rejuvenation Mask, Nefeli Intensive Daytime Skin Brightening Cream, Nefeli Intensive Nighttime Skin Brightening Cream

2. Spleen and Stomach Qi Deficiency

Symptoms manifested include low energy, indigestion, bloating and gas, loose stool or diarrhea, light-brown color spots on face, weak and slippery pulse, white/thick teeth-marked tongue.

TCM Root Treatment:

- Acupuncture: REN12, REN6, ST36, SP6, with moxa
- Herbal Treatment: Bu Zhong Yi Qi Tang (tonify middle decoction), Lu Jun Zi Tang (Six Gentlemen decoction), Nefeli Complete Balance, Nefeli Bright Complexion
- Food Therapy Suggestions: lotus root (powder), yiyi ren (coix seed), yam, orange peel, Chinese dates
- Topical Application: Nefeli Facial Rejuvenation Mask, Nefeli Intensive Daytime Skin Brightening Cream, Nefeli Intensive Nighttime Skin Brightening Cream

3. Liver and Kidney Yin Deficiency

The same analysis applies here as for liver and kidney yin deficiency causing dark eye circles. The deficiency can also cause facial discolorations. The discoloration and spotting usually are dark gray in color.

TCM Root Treatment:

- Acupuncture: REN4, KI3, LIV3, SP6

- Herbal Treatment: Nefeli Complete Balance, Nefeli Bright Complexion
- Herbal Treatment: Nefeli Total Eye Care, Nefeli Eye Refreshing Mask

- Food Therapy Recommendation: pear, sea cucumber, tremela, walnuts, mulberry, honey
- Topical Application: Nefeli Facial Rejuvenation Mask, Nefeli Intensive Daytime Skin Brightening Cream, Nefeli Intensive Nighttime Skin Brightening Cream

4. Yang Blockage with Blood Stasis

This type of facial discoloration and dark spots are usually dark and bluish in color accompanied by yang deficiency conditions, such as feeling cold in the limbs, bluish color on face and lips, a light and slow pulse, a bluish tongue with white coating.

TCM Root Treatment:

- Acupuncture: DU4, UB23, UB17, ST36, SP10
- Herbal Treatment: Tao Huang Si Wu Tang (modified according to patient's specific conditions), Nefeli Complete Balance, Nefeli Bright Complexion
- Food Therapy Suggestions: lotus seed, hawthrone berry, tomato, turnip, cilantro, cabbage, black fungus.
- Topical Application: Nefeli Facial Rejuvenating Mask, Nefeli Intensive Daytime Skin Brightening Cream, Nefeli Intensive Nighttime Skin Brightening Cream

Branch Treatment:

GB14, SI18, Tan Yang, ST7, GB20. Also, locate Ashi point inside discolored area.

CASE STUDY

A 58-year-old woman complains of facial discoloration and dark spots on her forehead and cheek area. Other signs and symptoms: patient went through her menopause several years ago. She had endometriosis before her period stopped. During the menopause period, her physician had prescribed her hormone replacement therapy, which she stopped about two years earlier. According to her, her dark spots started at about eight years earlier and progressed into dark discoloration spreading from her forehead first, then down to both cheeks. The shape of the discoloration looked like a butterfly. She had been suffering from insomnia, and body fatigue. Emotional stress always made the discoloration worse, as did sun exposure. She had been using over-the-counter anti-dark-spot creams, along with acid peels from time to time, to get rid of the discolorations. Nothing seemed to work. Her mouth was constantly dry. Hot flashes and night sweats were less recently but were still not totally gone. Her pulse was slightly fast, yet weak in Guan and Chi (kidney and liver) positions. Her tongue was red and slightly dry.

TCM Diagnosis:

Local blood stagnation with kidney yin deficiency and liver qi stagnation.

Her hot flashes and night sweats as well insomnia suggest her kidney yin deficiency. This deficiency causes congealed blood flow. Over a long time, yin deficiency burns the yin fruits causing heat and dryness, which further depletes the yin and causes yin blood to stagnant in the channel. Therefore, dark discoloration occurs in the facial area. Facial discolorations were worse, which points to her stagnated liver qi.

TCM Treatment Principle:

Tonify kidney yin, sooth liver qi, calm the spirit, promote local qi and blood flow, expel blood stasis, improve facial complexion.

TCM Treatment:

- Acupuncture Root Treatment: KI3, LIV3, SP10, SP6, LI11
- Acupuncture Branch Treatment: Ashi points (where the discoloration and dark spots are), Tai Yang, GB14, SI18

KI3 and LIV3 are both yuan source points of the kidney and liver system. They tonify kidney yin, build up liver yin blood, and clear deficiency heat. SP10 moves blood to the facial area. SP6 regulates three-yin channel and works as hormonal points. LI11 cools the blood and sends energy to the facial area.

During the treatment, KI3 and LIV3 were supplemented, while SP6, SP10, and LI11 were reduced.

- Acupuncture Branch Treatment: Ashi points (where the discoloration and dark spots are), Tai Yang, GB14, SI18
- Herbal Treatment: Dan Zhi Yiao Yao Wan (Peony and Garginia Wondering Powder), Nefeli Complete Balance, Nefeli Bright Complexion

- Food Therapy Suggestions: Chinese cabbage, white turnip, fresh or dried persimmon, fresh lemon, strawberries, tomatoes
- Topical Application: Nefeli Facial Rejuvenation Mask, Nefeli Intensive Daytime Skin Brightening Cream, Nefeli Intensive Nighttime Skin Brightening Cream"

Discolored area on her face immediately lessened while the needles were still on her face. Including all modalities she was recommended, after 10 treatments, 50 percent of the facial condition was improved.

21.5 Contraindications and Cautions for Facial Acupuncture Rejuvenation

There are contraindications associated with facial rejuvenation treatments. Practicioner must first rule out those patients who are not candidates for the facial rejuvenation treatment protocol:

- Do not treat infected, cut, or irritated skin.
- Do not treat very weak patients with severe qi and blood deficiencies.
- Do not treat patients with extreme stress or tension.
- Do not treat patients with extreme hunger, fatigue, sweating, diarrhea, hemorrhage, or bleeding.
- Pregnant patients may be lightly needled on the face. However, do not needle the contraindicated pregnancy points on the body.
- Do not treat patients with contagious skin diseases.
- Always avoid needling blood vessels.

- Diabetic patients may not be treated for facial rejuvenation.
- Do not needle hemophiliacs.
- Patients on Coumadin should be warned of bruising and must sign a prior consent form.
- Do not treat patients with severe migraines.

There are certain situations in which the practitioner should take extreme caution in their treatments.
- Always take caution in treating patients with extremely deficient body constitutions.
- If dizziness occurs after treatment:
  - Take needles out immediately.
  - Have the patient lower the head and raise the feet.
  - Loosen clothes and have the patient rest.
  - Offer the patient some hot water to drink.
  - For extreme dizziness, acupressure on DU26 and PC6; or moxa on REN 4 and REN 6.
- Always needle the body points first and the face points afterward. Then remove the needles from the face first and then from the body

Part II
Ping Zhang's Advanced Techniques
for Facial Rejuvenation

Section 8
Advanced Topics for Facial Rejuvenation

Traditional Chinese Medicine must be a continually developing and refined therapeutic practice. It is my belief that we, as TCM practitioners, must always strive to push our practices to a higher level by continuing to learn new treatment modalities and protocols. This is why I share with you my experience with TCM facial rejuvenation treatment modalities. I hope you will be interested in adding some of these techniques to your practice for the benefit of your patients.

The specific treatment protocols for different facial concerns that I have developed come from my many years of research study, advanced training, teaching, and clinic experience. These protocols include various modalities, including acupuncture, acupressure, herbal formulas, and qi gong, combined with the use of 100% natural herbal-based masks and creams to maximally benefit the treatment results. These protocols have worked very well for me and the participants who have taken my TCM facelift seminars. I am confident that they will work for you.

Chapter 22
Support Collagen Production for Wrinkles

22.1 Acupuncture/Acupressure Treatment

Acupressure:

Refer to the protocols in Chapter 12.

Acupuncture:

Facial Points:
- Tian Mu – 1 cun above Yin Tang. It is a point I commonly use for lifting the forehead and wrinkles in the forehead.
- SI18 – located under the lower board of zygomatic bone, in line with the outer canthus of the eye. This point strongly promotes qi and blood flow in the facial area.
- ST4 – clears wind from face; lifts and smoothes wrinkles around the mouth

- REN24 – reduces swelling of the face; promotes circulation of qi and blood

Figure 22.1 (See page.259) illustrates the combination of the above points.
Ashi Point – Choose a point in the center of wrinkles. Enter a needle straight into this center point (or deepest part of the wrinkle). Then using two needles, enter one needle from one end of wrinkle, threading towards the center, and enter the other from the other side of the wrinkle and threading toward the center.

Body Points:
Choose points from the yang ming and UB channels. The yang ming channel is full of qi and blood; activating them can readily send nutrients to the facial area. The UB channel back shu points connect to corresponding organ systems. Theese points regulate the internal organ system and stimulate healthy functioning of the skin. If you stimulate the yang ming and UB channels together, the skin will be nourished, and become more vibrant, smoother, and tighter.

Alternate 2 to 3 pairs of points from the following during each treatment.

- ST36 – lower He Sea point of the stomach yang ming channel. This point tonifies center body energy and supports a healthy immune system. It has strong anti-aging effects. It benefits the complexion and smoothes wrinkles. Enter needle perpendicularly and retain needle for 20 minutes. Supplement stimulation 3 times during the treatment.

- ST39 – lower He Sea point of the small intestine channel. This point firms the skin and nourishes dry skin. Enter the needle perpendicularly and retain needle for 20 minutes. Supplement stimulation three times during the treatment.
- ST41 – Stimulating this point can send energy toward the facial area. It clears heat from the face, reduces swelling of the face, and promotes skin healing in the face. Enter the needle upward at a 45-degree angle and retain needle for 20 minutes.
- LI9, LI10 – very effective points that promote qi and blood flow to the face, thus supporting healthy cell renewal of the skin. Choose one point at a time. Search for the more tender point and enter needle 45 degrees upward. Retain needle for 20 minutes. Supplement stimulation 3 times during the treatment.
- SP6 – three-yin intersection. This point tonifies kidney, liver, and spleen organ system and clears away damp heat. It is a major point used for anti-aging/anti-wrinkle purposes. Enter the needle at a 45-degree angle. Supplementally stimulate the needle 3 times during the treatment.
- SP10 – tonifies, detoxifies and promotes blood flow of the body so skin gets cleansed and rejuvenated at the same time. Enter the needle perpendicularly up to 1 cun. Supplement stimulation 3 times during the treatment.

Ear Points:

Heart, kidney, lung, face, Pi Zhi Xia (near the brain point), internal secretion. Use needles or ear seeds.

Adding the following procedure every other time during the treatment:
- Use finger stimulation from DU14 to DU2. Repeat up and down 5 times until the skin is red.
- Needle the following points: UB13, UB15, UB17, UB20, UB22, UB23.

22.2 Herbal Treatment

- Nefeli Wrinkle Smoother
- Nefeli Complete Balance
- Ren Sheng Yang Rong Wan
- Liu Wei Di Huang Wan

22.3 Moxa

REN4, REN6, REN8, REN12, ST36, Zhu Ming Guan – (Make a triangle with the line from REN12 to the left nipple as baseline, going outward the vertex. To find the point on the opposite side of the body, perform the same operation.) Each time, chose two points from the above points.

22.4 Jade Stick Massage

Jade as herbal for facial care has been used for thousands in China. In ancient times, herbalists crushed jade stone into fine powder and used it to exfoliate the face. Jade stick has also been used as a massage instrument for flattening the wrinkles and promoting healthy glow.

To use a jade stick for anti-wrinkle treatment, first, clean the patient's face. Then apply a thin layer of anti-wrinkle night cream on the face. (The author uses Nefeli Intensive Wrinkle Care Day Cream, which has a high concentration of pearls. Jade and pearls work very well together.) Hold the jade stick firmly, and follow the stroke and routine illustrated in Figure 22.2 (See page.259-262).

Because jade stick massage works well for wrinkles, it can be alternated with gua sha treatment.

22.5 Gua Sha

Perform gentle gua sha strokes on the wrinkle area. The gua sha strokes should only be performed in a one-way direction. Follow the same routine on the face as illustrated in Figure 22.3 (See page. 262- 264).

Make sure to use a good gua sha cream because gua sha helps the skin absorbs nutrients and detoxifies itself at the same time. Any natural, nutritional cream will work as gua sha cream. (The author uses Nefeli Intensive Wrinkle Care Night Cream for gha sha anti-wrinkle treatment.)

22.6 Food Therapy Suggestions

- Bird's nest
- Tremella
- E-Jiao
- Cherries

22.7 Topical Skin Care Applications

- Nefeli Intensive Wrinkle Care Day Cream
- Nefeli Intensive Wrinkle Care Night Cream
- Nefeli Facial Rejuvenating Mask

Chapter 23
Lymph Drainage

Lymph system energy flows with qi and blood, it is part of body fluids, and however, it functions as defensive part of qi system.

23.1 Acupuncture/Acupressure Treatment

Acupressure: Refer to protocols in Chapter 12.

Acupuncture:

Facial Points:
- DU26 – relaxes the face; calms the spirit; reduces facial swelling
- SJ21 – works as body water cleansing system
- ST7 – promotes local qi and blood flow; used as local motor point
- GB12 – clears heat; reduces facial swelling
- Yin Tang – clears heat; clears spirit

This point combination is illustrated in Figure 23.1 (See page. 265).

Body Points:

- Group 1:

  UB11, UB12, UB13, UB17, UB18, UB22. These UB channel points help lymph drainage from the internal body system.

- Group 2:
  - SJ5 – clears heat from the channels
  - DU14 – clears heat; relieves toxicity
  - LI4 – clears heat; reduces swelling of the face
  - SP10 – sea of blood; promotes blood flow; relieves toxicity
  - LI11 – clears heat from blood

Alternate these two groups in different treatments.

- Two-Triangle Method of the Back:
  - Triangle 1: DU 14 and UB 13, on both sides (bilaterally), form the first triangle on the upper back. Needle any points inside the triangle, including (a) any points on the edges of the triangle, (b) points on the passing channels, or (c) ashi points with any red or discolorations inside the triangle. Cupping in the triangle area is an alternative treatment. See the upper triangle shown in Figure 23.2 (See page. 265).
  - Triangle 2: DU5 and UB25 (bilaterally) form the second triangle on the lower back. Needle any points inside the triangle as prescribed for triangle 1. Cupping in the triangle area is an alternative

treatment. See the lower triangle shown in Fig. 23.2 (See page. 265).

Another alternative treatment to the two-triangle method is cupping Jia Ji points from UB12 to UB22.

Ear Points:
Lung, San Jiao, Kidney, Endocrine

23.2. Herbal Trearment

Nefeli Complete Balance

23.3 Gua Sha

Use gua sha technique on Jia Ji points from UB12 to UB22. Repeat 6–9 times until redness is seen on the back. A good gua sha skin application for lymph drainage purposes is safflower oil.

To check if there is Sha in the area that you decide to work on, simply use your thumb to press the area. If a red purple color appears and does not disappear right away, then you can consider using gua sha technique. Again, the stroke should be in a one-way direction.

23.4 Food Therapy Suggestions

Bitter melon, fresh luffa fruit, fresh dandelion, kiwi, green apple

Chapter 24
Lifting Sagging of the Face

24.1 Acupuncture/Acupressure Treatment

Acupressure:

Refer to protocols in Chapter 12.

Acupuncture:

Facial Points:
- DU20 – strongly promotes qi; lifts face
- ST8 – yang ming channel point that promotes qi and blood circulation
- UB8 – activates UB channel on the head; promotes local qi and blood flow; lifts the face
- REN23 – lifts chin area
- DU26 – strong point that opens energy (qi) flow in the face
- SJ17 – lifts sagging from the mandible area

- GB12 – reduces swelling; promotes lifting of the lower part of the face
- ST7 – promotes qi and blood flow to the face

Choose 3 or 4 points each time (See Fig.24.1 on page.265).

Body Points:
- ST36, GB34, UB40 – These leg yang He Sea (lower) points retain strong healing energy from yang organ system. When these points are activated, energy readily flows up to the facial area, supporting the nourishment of the facial muscles.
- ST36 – strongly tonifies qi and blood
- REN6 – strongly tonifies qi; lifts face

Ear Points:
Stomach, spleen, kidney

24.2 Herbal Treament

- Bu Zhong Yi Qi Tang (ginseng and astragalus combination)
- Nefeli Complete Balance

24.3 Moxa

REN4, REN6, REN12, ST36

24.4 Gua Sha

Gua sha protocol helps to detoxify the skin and lift the face. Figure.24.2 (pg.266-267) illustrates the gua sha protocol for sagging of the face. Make sure to apply anti-wrinkle/anti-sagging cream before starting the procedure.(Nefeli Intensive Wrinkle Care Night Cream is used in my practice.)

24.5 Jade Stick Massage

Jade stick massage not only works for wrinkle conditions, but also for lifting sagging of the face. Make sure to put on anti-wrinkle/anti-sagging cream before the massage. Figure 24.3 (pg. 267-269) demonstrates the protocol.

24.6 Food Therapy Suggestions

- Ginseng (contraindicated for patient's with high blood pressure)
- Yam
- Ge Gen (kudzu vine)
- Lamb

24.7 Topical Skin Care Application

- Nefeli Facial Rejuvenating Mask
- Nefeli Intensive Wrinkle Care Night Cream
- Nefeli Intensive Wrinkle Care Day Cream

Chapter 25
Facial Discoloration and Dark/Age Spots

25.1 Acupuncture/Acupressure Treatment

Acupressure:

Refer to protocols in Chapter 12.

Acupuncture:

Facial Points:
- ST7 – promotes local qi and blood flow to the face.
- SI18 – strong motor point that helps skin's detoxifying process
- Tai Yang – pulls all the yang energy from the face; promotes skin healing; releases toxic heat

Body Points:
- KI3 and LIV3 are both yan source points. They strongly tonify the organ system.
- LI11, SP10, SP6 are important points for promoting blood flow.

Ear Points (Shen Men):
Stomach, lung (upper and lower), large intestine, face, Jiong Ya Gou (lower blood pressure groove on back of ear) (See Fig. 25.1 on page. 269).

25.2 Herbal Treatment

Nefeli Bright Complexion

25.3 Gua Sha

Face Points:
Choose the local area where the discoloration is. Apply gua sha cream. Using the gua sha board, start from the center of the discolored area and spread outward in different directions with gentle force. Stop the procedure when slight redness is seen in the discolored area.

Always apply gua sha cream (facial brightening cream) before and during the procedure because this is the best time for the skin to absorb nutrients and release toxins. Use a gua sha cream that contains natural skin-brightening nutrients.

Besides the ashi points, the gua sha stroke on the face for dark/age spots should cover the following points: GB14, Tai Yang, SI18. Figure 25.2 (pg.269-270) illustrates the procedure.

Body Points:

- Upper back triangle area formed by DU14, UB13 (bilaterally): Perform gua sha strokes from upper to lower direction.
- LIV3: Scrape the point against the channel flow in one direction. Repeat 10 times.
- SP6, SP10: Scrape against the channel flow in one direction. Repeat 10 times for each point.
- LIV3 to LIV9: Scrape along the liver channel in the lower leg from LIV3 to LIV9 (all the way up). Repeat 10 times.

25.4 Food Therapy Suggestions

Winter melon, Chinese cabbage, white turnip, mulberry fruits, black fungus, Chinese dates

25.5 Topical Skin Care Application

- Nefeli Skin Brightening Wash
- Nefeli Intensive Day-Time Skin Brightening Cream
- Nefeli Intensive Night-Time Skin Brightening Cream
- Nefeli Facial Rejuvenating Mask

Chapter 26
Dark Eye Circles, Eye Bags and Puffiness of Eyes

26.1 Acupuncture/Acupressure Treatment

Acupressure:

Refer to protocols in Chapter 12.

Acupuncture:

Facial Points:
- UB2 – activates UB channel on the face; promotes qi and blood circulation in eye area
- Yu Yao – clears toxicity around eye area
- ST2 – a local Yang Ming point that moves qi and blood in eye area.
- GB14 – lift eyes; clears impurities from the face
- Tai Yang – clears heat; detoxifies local area

(See Fig. 26.1 on page.271)

Body Point:

- UB17, UB18, UB19, UB 23 – These UB channel points regulate internal organ system; promote qi and blood flow; and move blood stasis, including in the eye area.
- SP6, SP10 – Both points move blood. SP6 clears dampness and toxicity from the body, including dark eye circles, puffiness, and eye bags due to phlegm accumulations and blood stasis.
- KI3 – This yan source point tonifies kidney essence and kidney yin. Kidney essence and yin deficiency are major causes of dark eye circles.

For Eye Bags, add the following points:
- ST36 – tonify qi and blood; relieves dampness
- ST40 – transforms phlegm accumulation

For Dark Eye Circles, make sure to incorporate the following points for every treatment:
- ST36 – builds up qi and blood for the body
- SP10 – moves blood; cleanses blood
- SP6 – moves and tonifies blood; relieves dampness
- KI3 – This yan source point tonifies kidney essence and kidney yin.

26.2 Herbal Treatment

- Lui Wei Di Huang Wan
- Nefeli Eye Refresh

26.3: Gentle Gha Sha

Very light gua sha strokes can be applied to the eye area to promote local qi and blood flow and help treat dark eye circles, eye bags, and eye puffiness. Fig 26.2 illustrates the procedure (pg.271-272).

Caution: Because the eye area is very delicate, only light force is used, and each stroke is only repeated 6 times. Again, it is very important to apply eye cream before the gua sha procedure to protect the skin around the eyes and nourish the skin at the same time.

26.4 Gentle Jade Stick Massage

Gentle jade stick massage can also be applied (with eye cream) to the local area to help qi and blood flow. Fig 26.3 illustrates the steps (pg.272-273).

26.5 Food Therapy Suggestions

Black fungus, carrots, seaweeds, Chinese dates, wolfberries (gou qi zi), and lotus root

26.6 Topical Skin Care Application

- Nefeli Essential Eye Care Cream
- Nefeli Eye Rejuvenating Mask

Chapter 27
Flower Essence Skin Care

Using flower fragrance for beauty care is an ancient Chinese healing method. Chinese people have long recognized that the fragrance of certain flowers can help balance the body's yin and yang energy, relax the mind, and rejuvenate the skin. Note that the concept of flower essence in Traditional Chinese Medicine means using both the fragrance of the flower and its medical properties to heal the body. The ancient method uses less concentrated essences than today's commercial ready-to-use versions, yet they possess equal or greater healing properties.

TCM Flower Essence Body Care

For the most part, Traditional Chinese Medicine uses flower essences to balance the body's yin and yang energy through two properties:

1. Fragrance: The smell of an herb or flower is considered a very important aspect of its healing properties.

2. Healing agent: Another important aspect of the herb or flower is its therapeutic value as a medicinal plant. For example, if you chose to use rose essence oil for the facial concerns, it not only works as a hydrating agent to protect the skin from dryness, it also calms the mind and spirit while bringing a beautiful rosy luster to the face. All of these benefits are achieved by its fragrance, *and* by its qi and blood moving properties.

Ancient Chinese Flower Bathing Rituals

There are three types of bathing ritual traditions from ancient China:

1. Water Bath: This method uses just water and fresh flowers. The secret is the temperature of the water. Usually the water is very hot, but tolerable. Two baths present (usually made of wood) are drawn. One is for soaking the body; another smaller one, with even hotter water, is for soaking the feet. First, the bather soaks the body in the larger bath, to get the yang qi moving. With the body's energy channel opened up, the qi and blood flow helps cleanse the body. Afterward, the bather soaks the feet in the smaller, hotter bath. This is part of a "foot repairing" process, which is supervised by a specially trained foot specialist. He or she cleans and massages the bather's feet. Chinese healing theory believes aging starts from the feet and legs, so work on the feet (and legs) is very important for cleansing and tonifying the entire body, and calming the spirit.

2. Herbal Bath: An herbal bath is mainly used for treating body and skin conditions, though it also has anti-aging benefits. An herbal formula is prepared by the herbalist to treat a specific condition, or a traditional anti-aging and skin-body beautifying formula is used. The herbal formula is then soaked in cold water for couple of hours. Then it is boiled in the water for about 1 hour. The resulting herbal liquid is added to the bath water, sometimes in a measured amount if specified by the herbalist. For better results, the bath can be made very hot so a steam bath can be taken first. Then, when the water cools, the bather can soak in the bath. One can take a whole-body bath or a partial bath, depending on the specific condition.

3. "Dry" Bath: This waterless bath refers to the practice of An Mo massage. An An Mo practitioner uses his or her hands to massage the body's energy channel system in order to promote qi and blood flow, and to nourish essence, energy, and blood.

Some other ancient bath rituals using flower essences are the following:
- Using peach flower and snow water in the bath water to beautify and create a healthy glow on body and face
- Using seasonal fruit-bearing tree flowers and twigs in the bath to create a beautiful fragrance of the body and relieve body aches and relax the muscles
- Using flowers, like rosemary, and herbs, like nut grass, creating a beautiful fragrance to expel the "evil" from the body, and to calm and anchor the spirit

- Using wolfberries in the bath for longevity and disease prevention

Today, you, yourself do not have to collect the flower to prepare the essences, as they did in ancient times. There are many made ready-to-use flower essences on the market. You can simply purchase them, mix and match them as you choose, then use.

Individual Flower Essence for Different Skin Conditions

The following are brief descriptions of the flower essences that can safely be used in TCM herbal practice. You can use them in the bath for the patient, or add them to your self-made masks and washes to enhance treatment.

Lavender: heals sunburnt skin, soothes and relaxes the mind, and makes it easier to fall into a sound sleep.

Geranium: brings rosy colors to one's cheeks, adds luster to the skin, soothes and refreshes the brain, and relieves muscle tension.

Frankincense: retards the development of wrinkles, ensures a stable mental state and the preservation of vital energy, and dispels depression.

Petit Grain: relaxes and soothes sensitive skin and ensures clear, quick thinking. At the same time, it empowers the immune system.

Eucalyptus: keeps skin clean and soft and contributes to the mental concentration. At the same time, it clears away heat and toxic materials, removes dampness, and relieves itching.

Peppermint: helps skin cells discharge toxic materials and ensures clear, quick thinking. At the same time, it also eliminates swellings and removes blood stasis.

Rosemary: moisturizes and adds luster to the hair and improves memory. At the same time, it also helps the recovery of the body and mind.

Lemongrass: shrinks large pores and stimulates the spirit. At the same time, it removes unpleasant body odor and reduces swelling.

Sandalwood: moisturizes and softens dry skin, enhances mental power, and makes it easier to fall into sound sleep.

Sage: puts one in a pleasant and amiable mood and relieves women of their unpleasant feelings during their menstrual cycle.

Cedar Wood: prevents the brittle hair and split ends, eliminates dandruff, stabilizes the mental state, and speeds recovery of the body and mind.

Vetiver: shelters and protects sensitive skin, relieves sensitivity and numbness, and aids the circulation of vital energy and blood.

Flower Essence for TCM Facial Rejuvenation

Depending on the different formula of skin care being prepared, their usage can vary. A brief reference guide for the use of flower essences follows:

Warm Compress: Add 1 drop of the flower essence of your choice to 8 ounces of a steeped herbal wash. Choose from the above list of essences according to patient's skin conditions.

Herbal/Flower Essence Bath: This bath formula relaxes body, mind, and spirit, while enhancing skin beauty. Add 5 to 8 drops from 2 to 3 different kinds of flower essences to a full warm bathtub. Choose essences from the above list depending on the conditions of the patient.

Flower Essence Skin Cream: Add 1 to 2 drops of the flower essence of your choice, depending on your diagnosis of the patient. Mix with the available moisturizing cream.

Skin Care Spray: Mix 2 drops of 1 or 2 different flower essences from the above list to 100 ml herbal-based distilled water.

Part III

DIY Herbal Spa: TCM Needleless Facial Rejuvenation

Chapter 28
DIY Herbal Shop: TCM Needleless
Facial Rejuvenation

Often acupuncture facial rejuvenation clinic patients cannot receive acupuncture treatment due to a body condition, for example, patients on certain blood thinners, with high blood pressure, or in the early stages of pregnancy. However, such patients may still request a facial.

TCM has many modalities that apply to facial beauty. Instead of treating the patient with facial acupuncture, gentle facial acupressure, with the appropriate use of TCM herbal/food topical applications, can be performed. An herbal mask can be customized for different facial rejuvenation purposes, according to each individual's skin condition.

Caution: Before using any DIY herbal/food wash, exfoliate, mask, or cream, administer an allergy test on patient's inner wrist. Wait one day. If there is no allergic reaction (redness, swelling, etc.), then you may proceed to use them the product on your patient.

28.1 Making Herbal/Food Exfoliators

The following herbs/foods are commonly used in herbal exfoliation preparations: mung beans, wheat germs, rice germ, pearl, gypsum, jade.

Preparations:

For Oily Skin Type and Acne Care
Mix 1 Tablespoon mung bean powder with liquid made by chrysanthemums, make into thin past and exfoliate the face.

For Dry Skin and Discolored Skin
Combine 1 Tablespoon brown sugar with 1/4 teaspoon pearl powder and 1 teaspoon of olive oil. Mix well into a thin paste. Apply to the face as an exfoliator.

For Wrinkled and Aged Skin
Mix 1 Tablespoon wheat germ with 3 Tablespoons whole milk. Mix well into a thin paste. Apply to the face as an exfoliator.

Use Nefeli's Skin Brightening Wash as the base for customized exfoliator. Below are recommendations for varying the formula to address specific conditions:
- Add pearl powder for wrinkled skin.
- Add mung bean powder for discolored skin.
- Add brown sugar for dry skin.
- Add Da Huang (rhubarb) powder for acne conditions.

28.2 Making Herbal/Food Facial Masks
For Different Skin Types

Preparations:
For Dry Skin

Mix 15g of Xing Ren powder with 30g of Gua Lou powder, 1-1/2 teaspoons of soy powder (or soy protein), 1 teaspoon of honey, and 1 teaspoon of olive oil. Mix well. Apply the formula as a mask upon a clean face. Wait for 15 minutes, and then wash off.

For Oily Skin

Mix 1/2 teaspoon of chrysanthemum powder with 2 teaspoons of mung bean powder and 1 piece of 1x1x1 inch cube of tofu (soybean curd). Blend with 2 teaspoons of water. Apply the formula as a mask upon a clean face. Wait for 15 minutes, and then wash off.

For Sensitive Skin

Mix 1/2 teaspoon fresh aloe juice with 1/4 teaspoon chrysanthemum powder, and 1/4 teaspoon of pearl powder. Apply the formula as a mask upon a clean face. Wait 15 minutes, and then wash off.

For Combination Skin

Apply an oily-skin mask to the "T" zone area. Apply a dry-skin mask to the other areas.

28.3. Making Herbal/Food Masks
For Special Skin Conditions

Preparations:

For Wrinkled/Aged Skin and Sagging of Face

- **Fresh Luffa and Cucumber Mask:** Mix equal amounts of fresh luffa and cucumber. Blend the mix with 1/2 teaspoon pearl powder, 1/2 teaspoon honey (or 1/4 teaspoon of royal jelly), and 1 egg white (soaked in grain alcohol for 10 days). After into paste, apply upon a clean face. Wait 20 minutes, and then wash off.

- **Ginkgo Nut Mask:** Crush unshelled Ginkgo nuts into a paste. Add some water if necessary. Apply directly onto face. Wait 15 minutes and rinse off. Repeat daily.

- **Pig's Foot Mask:** Cut about a pound of pig's foot into small pieces. Boil the pig's foot in 64 ounces (8 cups) of water for about 2 hours, or until about a cup of liquid remains. Take out the meat and put just the soup in the refrigerator, where it will form a gelatin. Use as a regular mask by applying a portion onto the face at night and washing off the next morning.

  If using a pressure cooker, use 45 ounces of water with a pound of cut-up pig's foot. Bring to a boil, then mid-boil for 25 minutes. Follow the rest of the instructions as normal.

- **Chestnut Shell Mask:** Collect about 1 gram of the inner skin of the chestnut shell. Crush and mix with 2 teaspoons of organic honey. Apply upon a clean face at night, and wash off in the morning.

- **Banana and Strawberry Mask:** Blend 1/4 banana and 3 strawberries. Apply the mixture to the face for 15 minutes. Wash clean.

For Discolored, Dull Complexion/ Dark/ /Age Spotted Skin
- **Fu Ling Mask:** Take equal amounts of Fu Ling, Dong Gua Ren, Yi Yi Ren and mix with warm water. Apply to a clean face and wait for 15 minutes. Then wash off.
- **Eggplant Rub:** Cut off a good-size portion of fresh raw eggplant and rub the outside part around the face until the skin gets a little red. Then rinse.
- **Winter Melon Mask:** Mash the outside part of a winter melon (or crush 1/2 cup of winter melon seeds) and rub onto the face. Leave on for 20 minutes, then rinse off.
- **Egg in White Grain Alcohol:** Soak 7 eggs in 500 grams of grain alcohol and store in a tightly sealed jar for 7 days. Open and stir one of the eggs each day and apply onto the face for a few minutes, then wash off. Repeat daily for one week.
- **Luffa, Cucumber and Tomato Mask:** Juice together one fresh luffa, one cucumber, and one tomato. Drink half and use the rest as a topical mask. Rub some onto the face, and then wash off.
- **Persimmon Leaf Mask:** Look for persimmons with leaves still attached, or ask for persimmon leaf at a Chinese market. Dry the leaves and then crush them into a powder. Blend 50 grams of the dried persimmon leaf powder and mix with olive oil to form a sticky mask. Apply onto the spotted or discolored part of the face and leave on overnight. Wash away in the morning.

Repeat every night for at least two weeks, but not more than a month.

- **Cilantro Wash:** Wash and boil several stalks of fresh cilantro in 6 ounces of water for a couple of minutes, then use the juice to wash the face.

For Dark Eye Circles and Eye Bags

- **Promoting Circulation Mask:** Mix equal amounts of the following: safflower, Choung Xiong, Tao Ren, Xiong Ren, honey. Mix all the ingredients into a thin paste. Apply to eye area, but avoid touching the eyes. Wait for 15 minutes, and then wash off.
- **Chrysanthemum Flower Wash:** This wash is for dark eye circles and eye bags. Add 6 grams of chrysanthemum flowers to 6 ounces of boiling water. Let steep for 10 minutes in the pan. Then transfer to a bowl and let cool. Soak a hand towel in the warm "tea," and place the towel over both the eyes for 1 minute. Then resoak the towel and repeat. Repeat 5 times.
- **Sesame Seed Oil Mask:** This mask is used for eye bags. Simply apply sesame seed oil around the eyes before going to bed, and wash off in the morning. The best way to apply the oil is to dip a warm hard-boiled egg (with shell on) into the oil and then massage both eye areas with the egg.
- **Persimmon Peel Mask:** Peel the skin off a fresh, ripe persimmon and apply the peeled skin to the eye bags. Avoid touching the inside of the eye. The peel should be moist enough to stick. Leave on for 20 minutes, and then wash off.

- **Potato or Apple Skin Mask:** Remove 2 pieces of skin from a raw potato or apple and apply onto each eye bag. Hold for 10 minutes, and then wash off.

Caution: It is possible that you may be allergic to any of the above-mentioned herb/food masks. Before using a formula on the face, test it on the inner wrist by applying a dab and waiting 24 hours. If an irritation occurs, discontinue the mask and try another. If no reaction occurs, feel free to use the formula.

28.4. Making Your Own Skin Creams

In ancient times, the traditional procedure for making a facial cream used animal fat or wax as the cream base. They tended to be very greasy. Today with modern technology, the cream base can be made lightweight and easily absorbable. To make own your herbal/food cream, you can formulate your herbal mixture or choose your flower essence first; then mix to a cream base.

However, if you are interested in exploring the more advanced treatment and customized personal care, it is always possible to use self-made creams by adding herbal extracts to existing creams. For example, it is possible to use Nefeli's skin care formulas as a cream base for a self-made formula designed to treat a specific skin condition. The added herbal extracts serve two purposes: First, they more accurately treat different skin types affected by seasonal factors. For example, normal skin may become dry during the winter. Second, they promote deep skin healing for different kinds of skin conditions.

Preparations:

For Wrinkled/Aged Skin

Use Nefeli Intensive Wrinkle Care Night Cream as a cream base. Add extra herbal formula depending the patient's individual skin conditions.

- For wrinkled/aged, dry skin; add herbal extract of cactus and seaweed.
- For wrinkled/aged, oily skin, add herbal extracts of chrysanthemum.
- For wrinkled/aged, sensitive skin, add herbal extract of green tea.
- For severe wrinkles and sagging, add more ginseng and astragalus extracts.

For Facial Discolorations, Dark/Age Spots

- Use Nefeli Intensive Nighttime Skin Brightening Cream as a cream base. Add extra herbal formula depending the patient's individual skin conditions.
- For dry skin, add herbal extract of cactus and liquorice.
- For oily skin, add herbal extracts of chrysanthemum.
- For sensitive skin, add herbal extract of safflower.
- For severe discoloration, dark/age spots, add pearl powder and more herbal extract of winter melon.

For Eye Concerns

- Use Nefeli Essential Eye Care Cream as cream base.

- For severe dark circles, add herbal extracts of Zhi Cao and safflower.
- For eye bags, add herbal extract of seaweeds and/or ivy.

Chapter 29
Step-by-Step Procedures
For TCM Spa Facial Rejuvenation

In this chapter, I share my TCM spa facial rejuvenation procedures. I hope this will help you to build a spa that combines all the possible healing modalities for the benefit of the patients. You may already have very good protocols in your clinic. If that is the case, I hope you will learn something different and incorporate some of the techniques you find helpful to integrate your current practice.

Following are step-by-step instructions for acupuncture, acupressure, and herbal (needleless) facial rejuvenation protocols:

Step 1. Clean the face: Thoroughly clean the face with Nefeli's Skin Brightening Wash. This is the initial activating step for skin healing.

Step 2. Exfoliate the face: Use self-made exfoliators according to patient's skin type. Wash the face clean to prepare for acupuncture.

Step 3: Facial acupuncture: Comply with clean needle technique during the procedure. Follow the routine as discussed in this book. Acupuncture treatment should take less than 35 minutes.

If cupping is necessary, then perform the procedure after the needling. Leave cups on skin for about 5 minutes. **Note:** If only acupressure facelift protocol is performed, skip this step.

Step 4: Facial acupressure: Perform acupressure protocol on the face to promote deep qi and blood flow to the muscle and skin layer, rejuvenate the skin cells, and improve the skin's collagen production. Make sure to use a good herbal-based cream. Follow the acupressure facial rejuvenation procedures as mentioned in this book. Use the following massage creams during the procedure:

- For wrinkles and sagging face: Use a self-made massage cream or Nefeli Intensive Wrinkle Care Night Cream.
- For discolorations and dark/age spots: Use a self-made massage cream or Nefeli Intensive Nighttime Skin Brightening Cream.

The entire acupressure procedure should take less than 10 minutes.

Step 5: Gua sha or jade stick massage: Both gua sha and jade stick massage are effective for all facial rejuvenation concerns. Use gua sha and jade stick massage alternately as separate treatments. Do not use them during the same treatment session.

Apply the gua sha protocols appropriate for the patient's skin conditions. It is especially effective for treating dull complexion, dark/age spots, and deep wrinkles. Make sure to use an effective gua sha cream or oil, either self-made or Nefeli Intensive Nighttime Skin Brightening Cream.

Use the jade stick massage protocols appropriate for the patient's conditions. Jade stick massage is especially effective for lifting sagging of the face and firm the skin.

It should take about 8 minutes to finish either gua sha or jade stick massage.

Step 6: Apply a self-made herb mask appropriate for the patient's skin condition, or use Nefeli Facial Rejuvenating Mask and Nefeli Eye Rejuvenating Mask. Make sure to use both together by applying the eye rejuvenating mask first and then the facial rejuvenating mask. Leave the masks on for 15 minutes, and then remove them.

Step 7: Finish by applying self-made skin cream or a Nefeli cream based on the patient's skin conditions.

Step 8: Perform qi gong exercises together with the patient (optional).

Step 9: Patient's home care plan for facial and body rejuvenation:
- **Herbal suggestions:** Choose a skin healing formula, or use the Nefeli line of herbal supplements, including facial, eye, and body concerns. If you decide to use the

Nefeli line of anti-aging herbal supplement, here are some suggestions:

- For body and mind and face, use Nefeli Complete Balance.
- For wrinkles and sagging of the face, use Nefeli Wrinkle Smoother.
- For dull complexion and dark/age spots, use Nefeli Bright Complexion.
- For eye concerns including dull eye vision, tired eyes, dark eye circles, eye bags, puffy eyes, fine lines around eyes, and claw's feet, use Nefeli Eye Refresh.
- For double chin due to overweight, use Nefeli Weight Management.
- If the patient's facial concerns are due to yin deficiency causing menopause, use Nefeli Menopause Soother.
- If the patient's facial concerns are due to seasonal allergies (dark eye circles and puffy eyes due to seasonal allergies, for example), use Nefeli Cold and Allergy Care.

- **Dietary suggestions:** Recommend to your patient skin healing foods (refer to the related chapters from this book) according to his or her skin conditions.
- **Qi gong exercise:** Perform qi gong exercise together with the patient (optional) at the first time. Patient should practice qi gong exercise once a day.
- **Topical skin application:** Suggest to your patient a pure, safe, natural skin care product that best fits his or

her skin conditions. If you choose to recommend the Nefeli natural herbal-based skin care line for your patient, you can follow these suggestions:

- For dull complexion and dark/age spots: Nefeli Skin Brightening series.
- For lifting sagging of the face and wrinkles: Nefeli Wrinkle/Aged Skin
- For dark eye circles, eye bags, puffy eyes, and fine lines around the eyes, including crow's feet: Nefeli Essential Eye Cream, Nefeli Facial Rejuvenating Mask, and Nefeli Eye Rejuvenating Mask
- For cellulite reduction and weight management: Nefeli Cellulite Cream
- For more sophisticated high-level skin care: Nefeli customized fresh Herbal Liquid Essence can be freely added to other creams for specific skin concerns.

- **Body and spirit rejuvenation:** Take a herbal/flower essence bath twice a week for body and face relaxation. Refer to the previous chapter for flower essence remedies.

Caution: When using any of self-made washes, masks, or creams, first administer a skin test for any allergic reactions. Simply apply a small portion on the patient's inner wrist and wait 24 hours. If an allergic reaction occurs, stop using it. If there is no allergic reaction, then feel free to use the product.

Appendix A

Acupressure Protocols - Picture Demonstrations

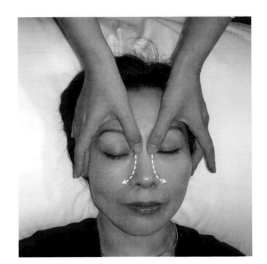

Fig. 12.1

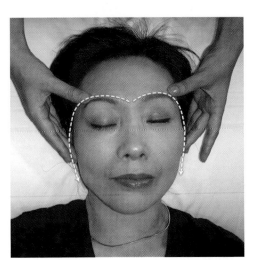

Fig. 12.2

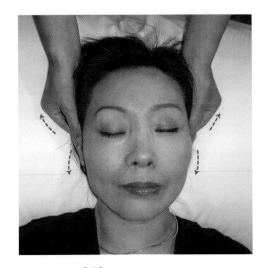

Fig. 12.3

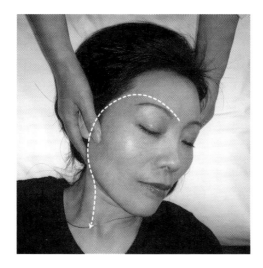

Fig. 12.4

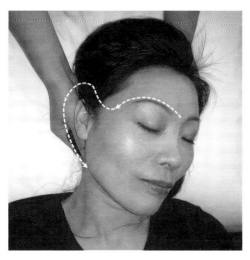

Fig. 12.5

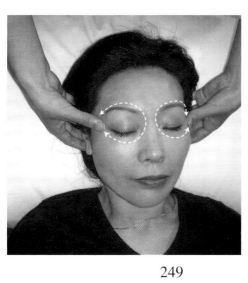

Fig. 12.6

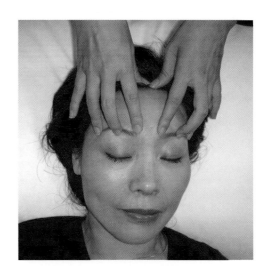

Fig. 12.7

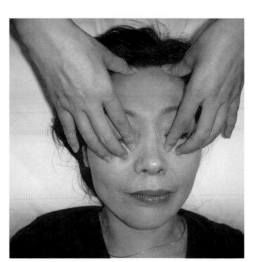

Fig. 12.8

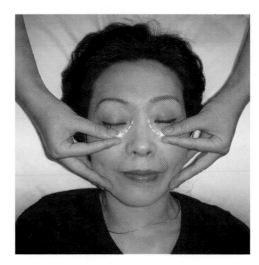

Fig. 12.9

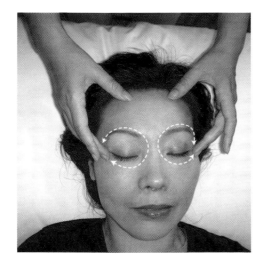

Fig. 12.10

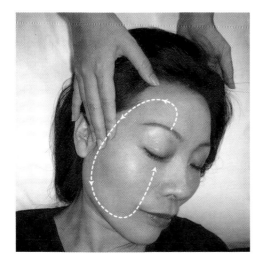

Fig. 12.11

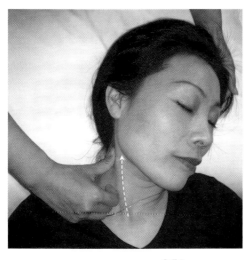

Fig. 12.12

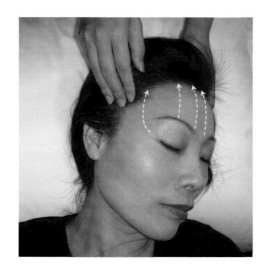

Fig. 12.13

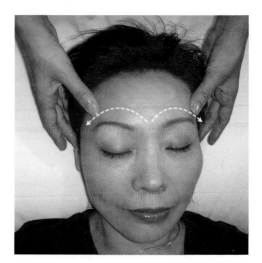

Fig. 12.14

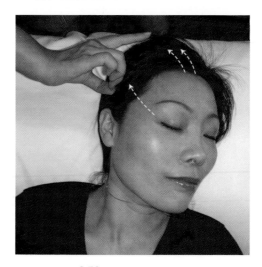

Fig. 12.15

Appendix B

Acupuncture, Gua Sha and Jade Stick Massage
- Picture Demonstrations

Cross friction Gua
Sha on vertical
wrinkle line
Fig. 19.1

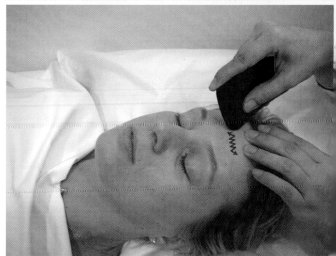

Cross friction Gua
Sha on horizontal
wrinkle line
Fig. 19.1

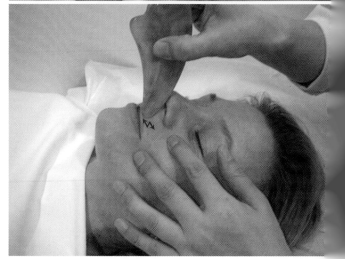

Cross lip line
friction Gua Sha
Fig. 19.1

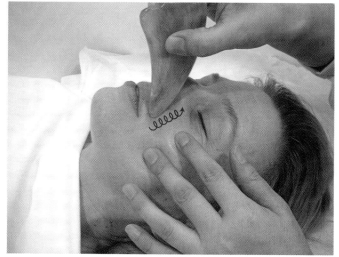

Spiral motion Gua Sha on nasolabial line

Fig. 19.1

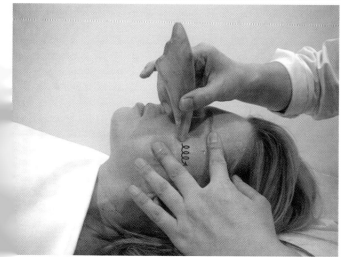

Spiral motion Gua Sha on claw's feet

Fig. 19.1

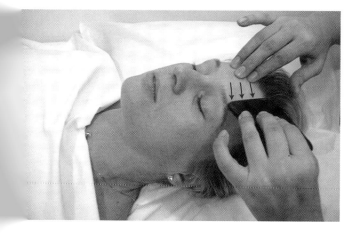

Fig. 19.2

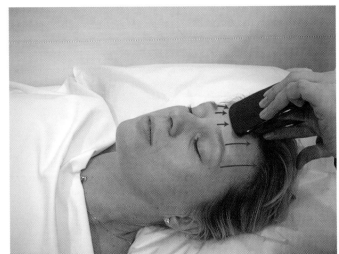

Fig. 19.3

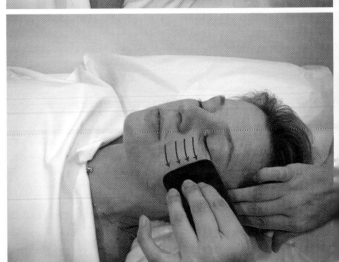

Fig. 19.4

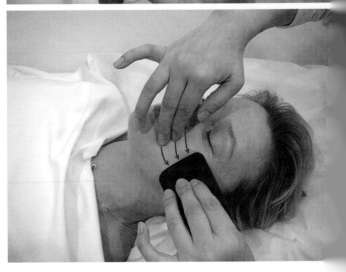

Fig. 19.5

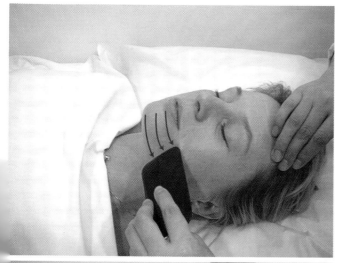

Fig. 19.6

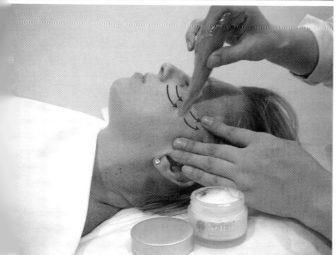

Fig. 19.7

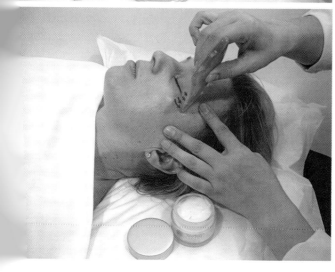

Fig. 19.8

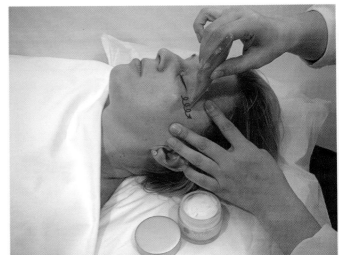

Fig. 19.9

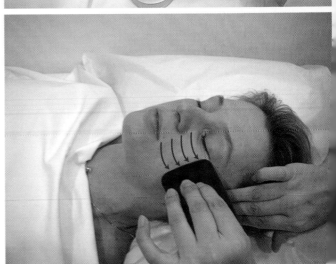

Fig. 19.10

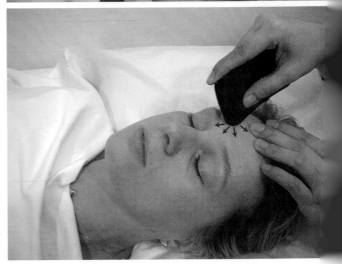

Fig. 19.11

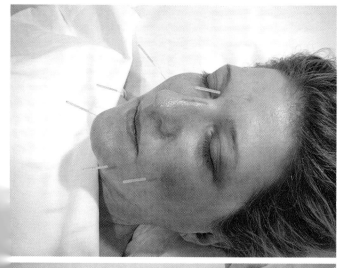

Fig. 22.1

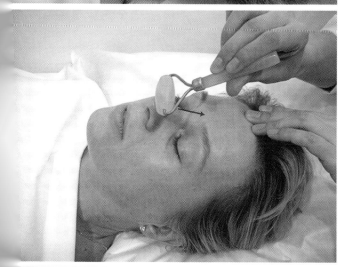

Fig. 22.2
Step-1

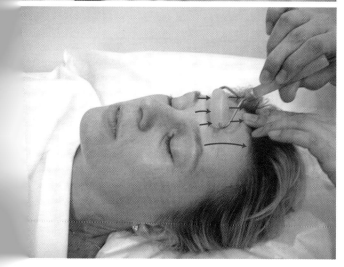

Fig. 22.2
Step-2

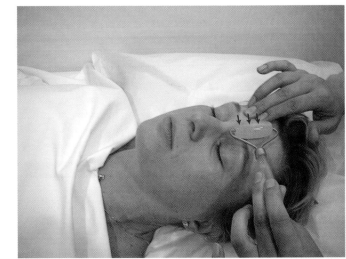

Fig. 22.2
Step-3

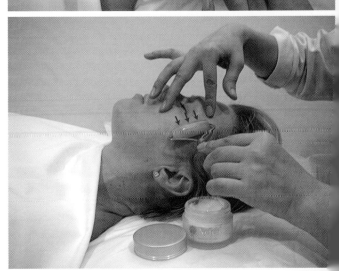

Fig. 22.2
Step-4

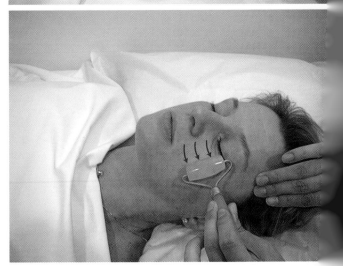

Fig. 22.2
Step-5

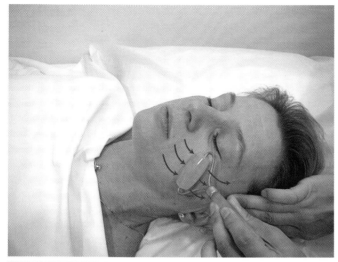

Fig. 22.2
Step-6

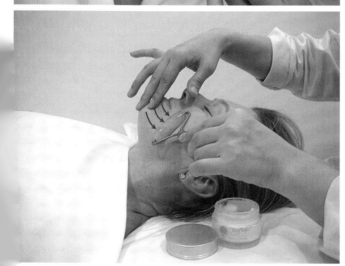

Fig. 22.2
Step-7

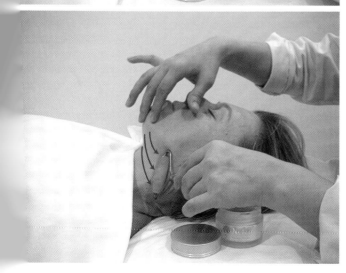

Fig. 22.2
Step-8

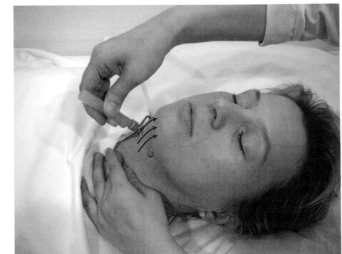

Fig. 22.2
Step-9

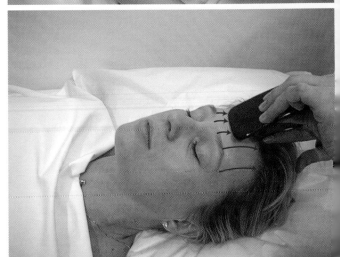

Fig. 22.3
Step-1

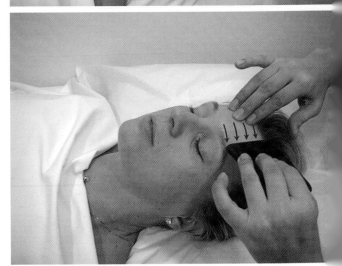

Fig. 22.3
Step-2

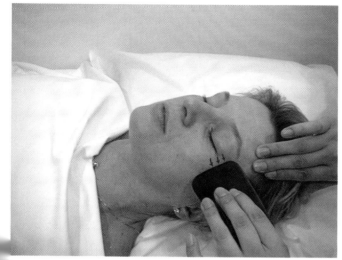

Fig. 22.3
Step-3

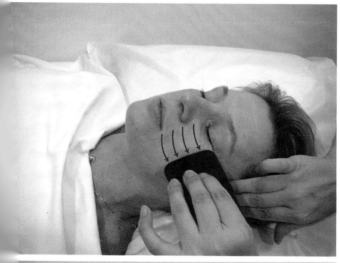

Fig. 22.3
Step-4

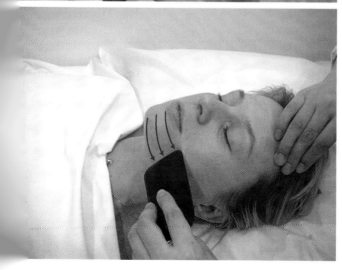

Fig. 22.3
Step-5

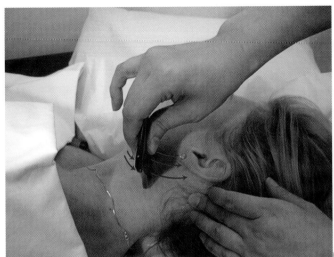

Fig. 22.3
Step-6

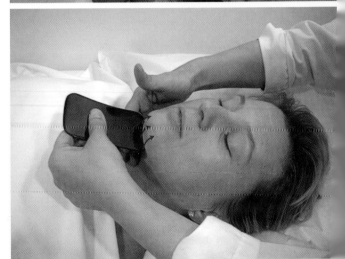

Fig. 22.3
Step-7

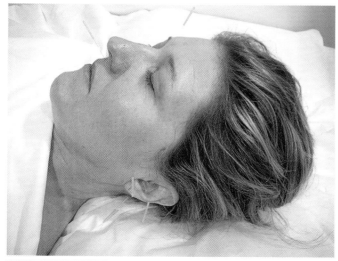

Fig. 23.1

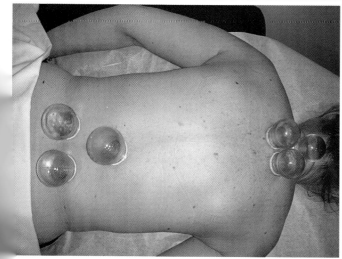

Cupping on upper and lower triangle

Fig. 23.2

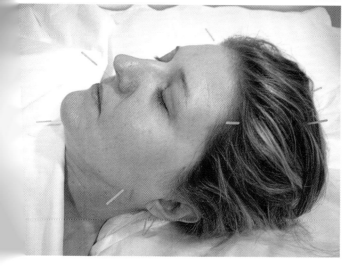

Fig. 24.1

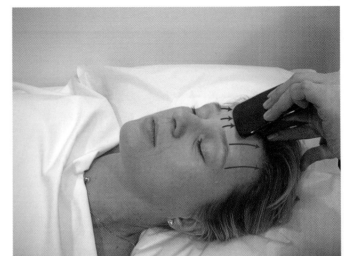

Fig. 24.2
Step-1

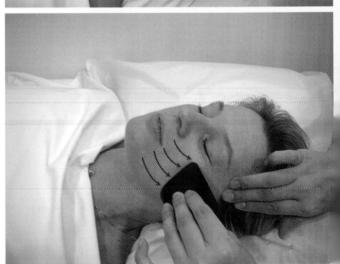

Fig. 24.2
Step-2

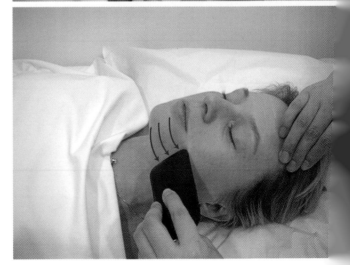

Fig. 24.2
Step-3

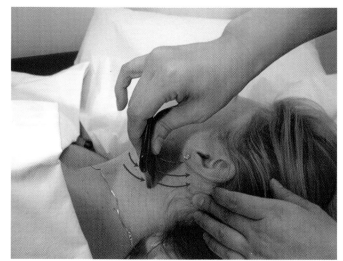

Fig. 24.2
Step-4

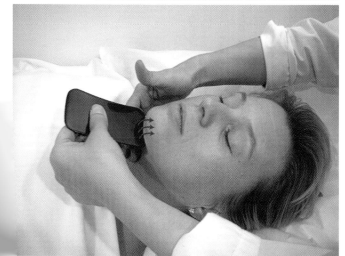

Fig. 24.2
Step-5

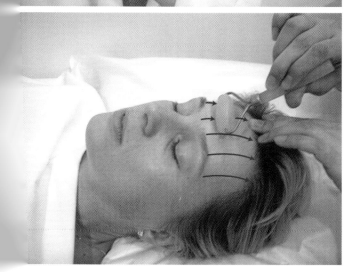

Fig. 24.3
Step-1

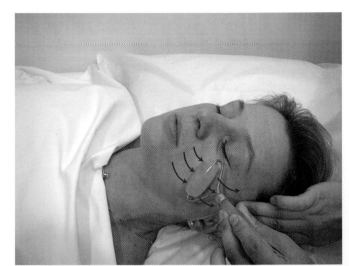

Fig. 24.3
Step-2

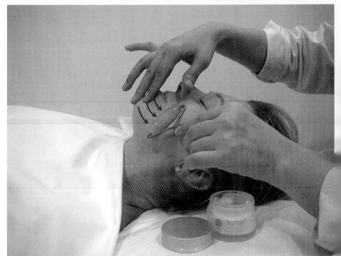

Fig. 24.3
Step-3

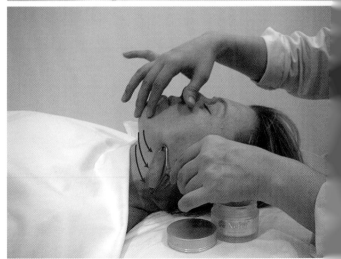

Fig. 24.3
Step 4 -

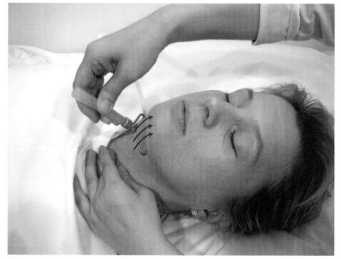

Fig. 24.3
Step-5

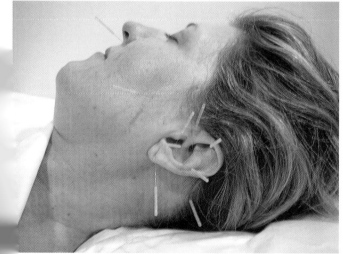

Fig. 25.1

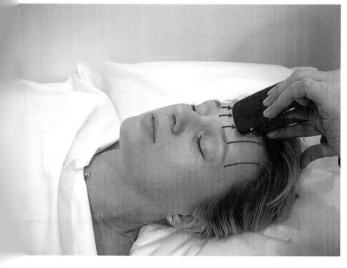

Fig. 25.2
Step-1

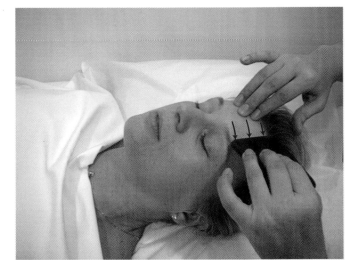

Fig. 25.2
Step-2

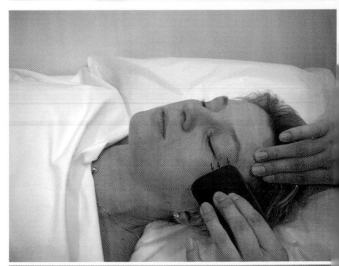

Fig. 25.2
Step-3

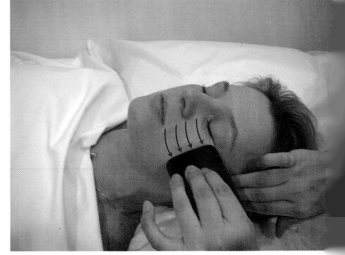

Fig. 25.2
Step-4

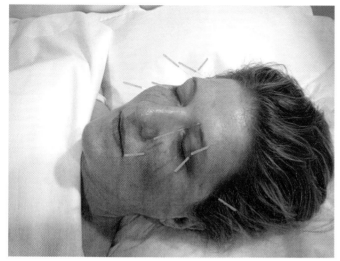

Fig. 26.1
Step-5

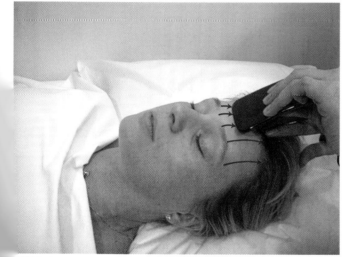

Fig. 26.2
Step-1

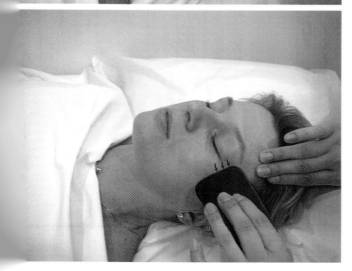

Fig. 26.2
Step-2

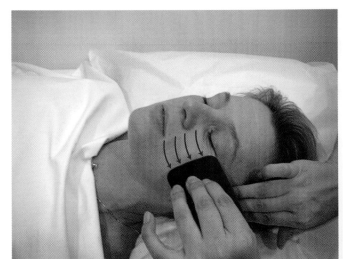

Fig. 26.2
Step-3

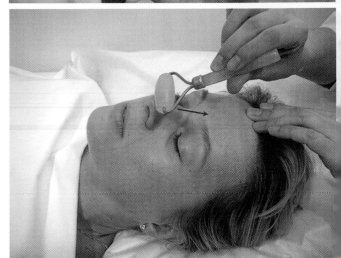

Fig. 26.3
Step-1

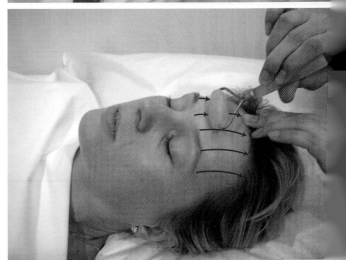

Fig. 26.3
Step-2

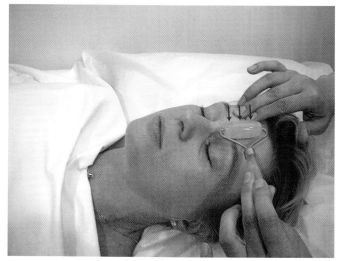

Fig. 26.3
Step-3

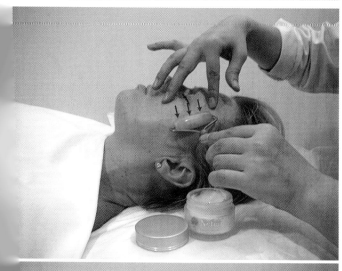

Fig. 26.3
Step-4

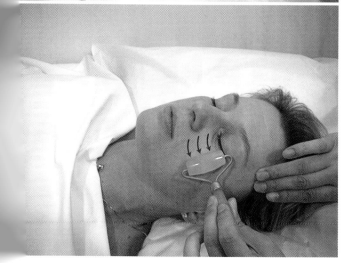

Fig. 26.3
Step-5

Traditional Chinese Medicine Facial Rejuvenation
Before and After Pictures

Ping Zhang's Needleless TCM
Facial Rejuvenation (30 day program)

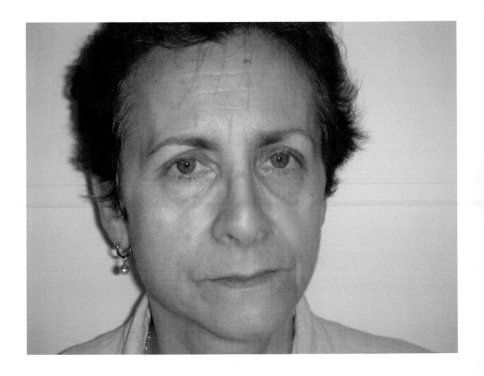

Before

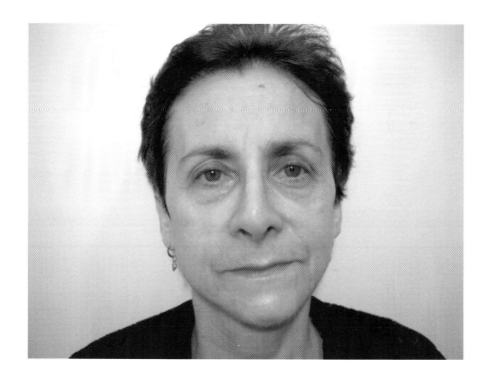

After

There is a significant lift from this woman's face. Her skin becomes more radiant and firm. Her jaw line is more defined. The appearance of forehead and frown wrinkles as well as nasolabial folds has been improved. Eyes are more lifted. Eye bags become smaller and less puffy.

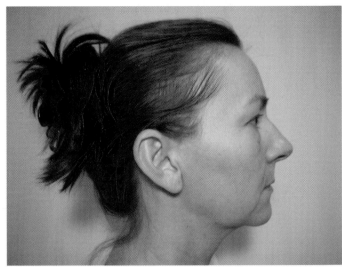

Before

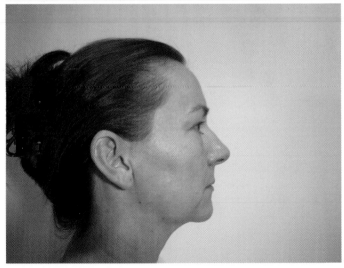

After

This woman's jaw is more defined and the appearance of her facial contour has been improved. Sagging appearance of the chin is lifted. Her eye bags are less puffy. Her nasola-bial line and the lines at the corner of her month become less deep

Bibliography

Chinese Herbal Medicine for Facial Beauty (*Zhong Yao Mei Rong Yong Yan*), Chinese edition. Sun Li Quan. Southern China Science and Technology University Press, 2003.

Classic of the Mountains and Seas (*San Hai Jing*), Chinese Edition. Warring States period (770–221 B.C.).

Divine Husbandman's Classic of the Materia Medica, (*Shen Nong Ben Cao Jing*), Chinese edition. Qin-Han dynasty (221–264 B.C.).

Encyclopedia of Traditional Chinese Medicine – Qi Gong Xue (*Zhong Gue Yi Xue Bai Ke Quan Shu – Qi Gong Xue*) Chinese edition. Shanghai Science and Technology Publishing House, 1982.

Ge, Hong. *Emergency Formulas in the Sleeve* (*Bei Ji Zhou Hou Fang*), Chinese edition. West Jin dynasty (265 A.D.).

Huang, Pu Mi. *Systemized Canon of Acupuncture and Moxibustion* (*Zhen Ju Jia Yi Jing*), Chinese edition. Jin dynasty, (282 A.D.).

Li, Shi Zhen. *Grand Materia Medica* (*Bei Cao Gang Mu*), Chinese edition. Liu, Heng Rou, ed. Ming dynasty (1578 A.D.). People's Health Publishing Press, 1995.

Lin, Juen Hua. *Practical Traditional Chinese Medicine for Rejuvenation* (*Lin Chuong Mei Rong Xue*), Chinese edition. China Medical Science and Technology Publishing House, 2004.

Shi, Xua Ming. *Traditional Chinese Medicine Encyclopedia* (*Zhong Yi Gong Mu*). Chinese edition. People's Journal Publishing House, 1992.

Sun, Si Mao. *Supplement to the Thousand Ducal Formulas* (*Qian Jin Yi Fang*), Chinese edition. Tang dynasty (618–907 A.D.).

Sun, Si Mao. *Thousand Ducat Formulas* (*Qian Yin Yao Feng*), Chinese Edition. Tang dynasty (618–907 A.D.).

Wang, Bin, ed. *Yellow Emperor's Inner Classic* (*Huang Di Nei Jing*). Consists 2 parts: *Spiritual Axis* (*Ling Shu*), Han dynasty (206 B.C.–20 A.D.); and *Plain Questions* (*Su Wen*), Tang dynasty. Chinese edition. Shanghai Ancient Text Publishing House, 1991.

Wang, Wei Yi. *The Life Promoting and Prevention Classic of Acupuncture and Moxibustion* (*Zhen Ju Zhi Shen Jing*), Chinese edition. (1220 A.D.).

Yang, Jia San. *Acupuncture Text Book* (*Shu Xue Xue*). Chinese edition. Shanghai Science and Technology Publishing House, 1987.

Yang, Ji Zhou. *Great Compendium of Acupuncture and Moxibustion* (*Zhen Ju Da Cheng*), Chinese edition. Ming dynasty (1601 A.D.).

Xiao, Ging Sheng. *Encyclopedia for Chinese Life Preservation and Prevention* (*Zhong Hua Yang Sheng Bao Jian Ci Hai*). Chinese Cultural and History Publishing House, 2003.

Zhang, Ping. *Anti-Aging Therapy: How to Clear Away Wrinkles and Rejuvenate Your Face.* Nefeli Corp., 2005.

283

About the Author

Ping Zhang is the president and founder of Nefeli Corporation. She holds a Ph.D. in Oriental Medicine, and is a New York State licensed acupuncturist and a national certified herbalist. Dr. Ping Zhang has more than 10 years of clinical experience in anti-aging Traditional Chinese Medicine (TCM).

As a pioneer in the field of anti-aging Traditional Chinese Medicine, she was the first to introduce and design a graduate – level course in TCM Facial Rejuvenation in the United Status.

She is the author of *Anti Aging Therapy*, where she introduced anti-aging Traditional Chinese Medicine to the American public. She also published a series of educational CDs on anti-aging therapy for healthcare professionals.

Dr. Ping Zhang is the creator of Nefeli, an anti-aging product line highlighting anti-aging nutritional herbal supplements and natural herbal- based skin care.

She represents the fourth generation of her family to practice Traditional Chinese Medicine. She is frequently interviewed as an expert in TCM and her unique natural herbal and skin care line has been featured in major news media channels and magazines, such as WABC-TV (Channel 7 Eyewitness News), WB11 (Channel 11 News), Newsday, Hartford Courant, Reuters News, World Journal (Chinese), Elle Magazine, Les Nouvelles Esthetiques, Public TV, Nikki Style Magazine, Healing Lifestyle and Spas, Today's Black Women, Elements Magazine, etc.

Dr. Ping Zhang is currently hosting her web radio program titled *Traditional Chinese Medicine with Dr.Ping* in Progressive Radio Network, , and continually teaches and lectures internationally for healthcare professionals while maintaining a high volume private practice in Port Washington, NY.